AF615633

Step by Step Guide to MESOTHERAPY

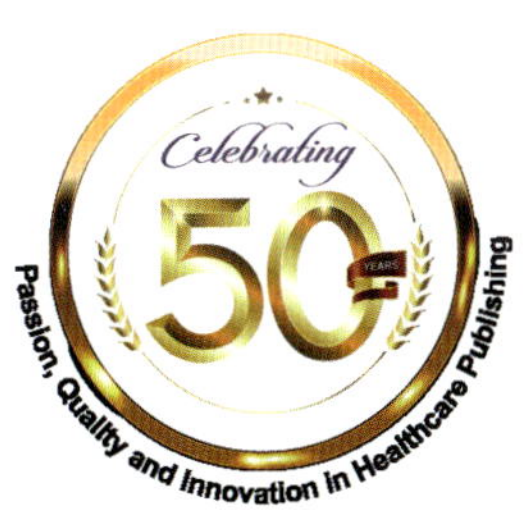

Step by Step Guide to MESOTHERAPY

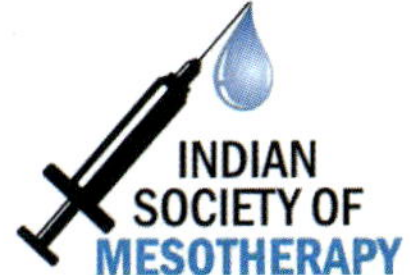

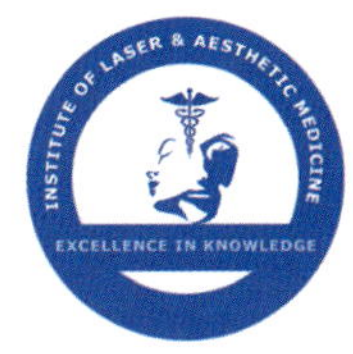

Jacques-Henri Coulon MD
Specialized in Homeopathy and Mesotherapy
General Practitioner, Homeopathy and Mesotherapy
Dampierre, France
President, Society of Mesotherapy of Franche-Comté

Co-author
Ajay Rana MD
Dermatologist and Aesthetic Physician
Founder and Director
Institute of Laser and Aesthetic Medicine (ILAMED)
New Delhi, India
President
Indian Society of Mesotherapy
Indian Society of Aesthetic Medicine

Foreword
Denis Laurens

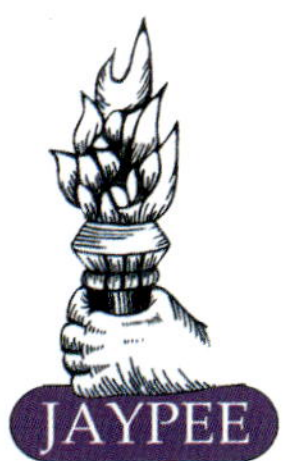

JAYPEE BROTHERS MEDICAL PUBLISHERS
The Health Sciences Publisher
New Delhi | London | Panama

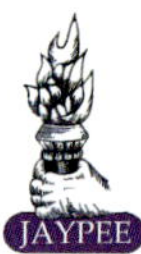

Jaypee Brothers Medical Publishers (P) Ltd

Headquarters

Jaypee Brothers Medical Publishers (P) Ltd
4838/24, Ansari Road, Daryaganj
New Delhi 110 002, India
Phone: +91-11-43574357
Fax: +91-11-43574314
Email: jaypee@jaypeebrothers.com

Overseas Offices

J.P. Medical Ltd
83 Victoria Street, London
SW1H 0HW (UK)
Phone: +44 20 3170 8910
Fax: +44 (0)20 3008 6180
Email: info@jpmedpub.com

Jaypee-Highlights Medical Publishers Inc
City of Knowledge, Bld. 235, 2nd Floor
Clayton, Panama City, Panama
Phone: +1 507-301-0496
Fax: +1 507-301-0499
Email: cservice@jphmedical.com

Jaypee Brothers Medical Publishers (P) Ltd
Bhotahity, Kathmandu, Nepal
Phone: +977-9741283608
Email: kathmandu@jaypeebrothers.com

Website: www.jaypeebrothers.com
Website: www.jaypeedigital.com

Step by Step Guide to Mesotherapy

First Edition: **2019**

ISBN: 978-93-5270-909-0

Printed at: Samrat Offset Pvt. Ltd.

Dedicated to

My beloved wife, Rosaline
who supported me with patience during this long work,
and to my three daughters, Anne, Elisabeth, and Mary.
In memory of my parents and grand parents.
A friendly thought for my collegues of the CERM of Franche -Comté,
and to my collegues of the French Society of Mesotherapy,
especially the Dr Jean-Marc Piumi, President of the SFM,
and Dr Denis Laurens, previous President
who helped me with attention and Friendship.
A special thank to the Dr Ajay Rana, co-author of the book,
Founder of the Indian Society of Mesotherapy,
with whom I have had a precious and constructive collaboration.
To end this dedication,
I have to say that this book is a special tribute
to the Dr Michel Pistor, Founder of Mesotherapy;
he taught me all I know now, and always with simplicity and wisdom;
he was a great physician and deserves a profound respect from me.

—Jacques-Henri Coulon

My wife—Anne,
my daughter—Olivia,
and
my parents—Janak and Netar

—Ajay Rana

FOREWORD

Mesotherapy, the French invention of Dr Michel Pistor in 1952, is now used by numerous doctors worldwide.

But to obtain better results, mesotherapy must be practiced with a great scientific rigor. In 16 countries, members of the International Society of Mesotherapy, the teaching of mesotherapy is dispensed by the International Course developed by Dr André Kaplan on the basis of the validated Interuniversity Diploma, and recognized by the French authorities.

This book of Dr Jacques-Henri Coulon and Dr Ajay Rana will be a precious help for all the mesotherapists who will be able to improve their knowledge and techniques.

This is the first time that a book handling indications and techniques of mesotherapy is published in English language.

The clinical pictures are clear, precise, and the protocols are very well-explained.

There is no doubt that this book will allow the progress of mesotherapy practice in the world.

Denis Laurens MD
President
French Society of Mesotherapy

PREFACE

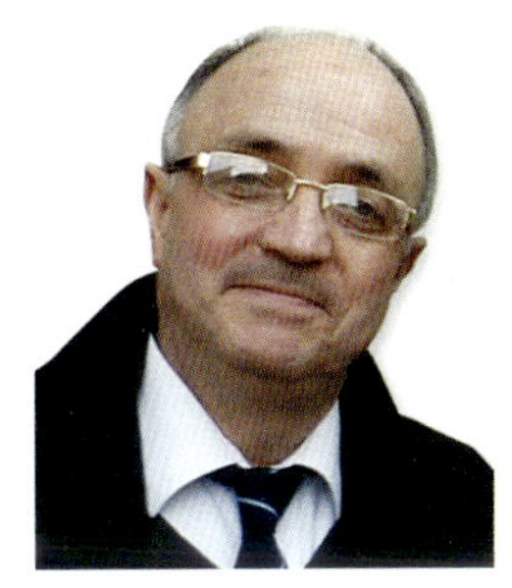

This book has no other aim than to provide to my young colleagues a practical and safe way to treat patients.

Mesotherapy is a wonderful technique which I used since 30 years, with constant and good results on several pathologies, especially in domains like rheumatology, sports injuries, pains, and vascular diseases.

I had the great chance to meet Dr Michel Pistor in the eighties; he was the conceptor of mesotherapy (1952), and taught me all about this technique and what could be treated. He founded the French Society of Mesotherapy in 1964; Centers of Research in Mesotherapy were created in France in 1981; and The International Society of Mesotherapy was created in 1984.

Mesotherapy has been officially recognized by the French Academy of Medicine in 1987 and a diploma is now necessary for the practice of mesotherapy in France.

I have taught mesotherapy in my own Society of Mesotherapy (CERM of Franche-Comté) for about 10 years, and I have presented my works in the French Congress of Mesotherapy in Paris (1985); those works were about the mesotherapy treatment of neurovegetative dystonia (100 cases).

I wrote the first book in 1987 "Comparated Stimulotherapies in Medical Practice", published in Paris (Maloine Editor), and in Brazil and Italy.

This book is based on my interest of associating three techniques: mesotherapy, acupuncture, and auriculotherapy.

Jacques-Henri Coulon

PREFACE

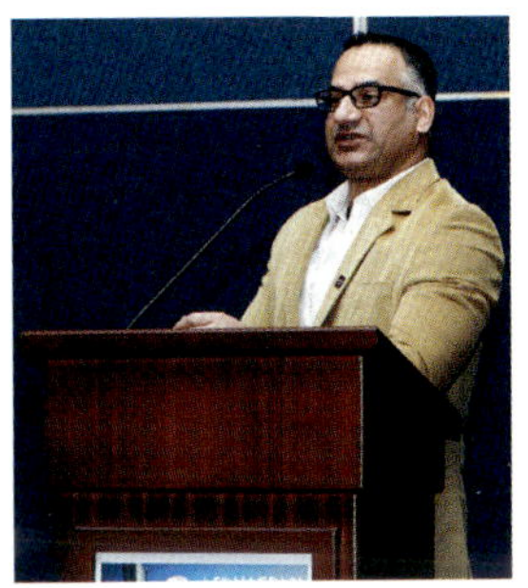

A new demographic and economic landscape in India has led to an increased pressure on healthcare managers and providers. Consequently, the Indian medical system is now characterized by the coexistence of various schemes designed to address the needs of an ever-increasing population.

Mesotherapy consists of injecting small quantities of potent medicine through needles over various points in the body, combining the power of allopathy with a soft mode of administration. It diminishes negative side effects of medicines for it is given at intervals through small dosages. Mesotherapy can benefit a huge number of patients.

The Indian Society of Mesotherapy (ISM) was later established under the aegis of the International Society of Mesotherapy (ISM) and the French Society of Mesotherapy (FSM) to promote mesotherapy in the Indian subcontinent. The ISM's mission is to promote research and teach medical practitioners clinical as well as esthetic aspects of Mesotherapy. Through its courses, practitioners in India gain comprehensive education and technical training in the evolving science of mesotherapy.

Now, we wish to pursue the integration of mesotherapy within the current medical system of India. Through exchanges and common studies, they pursue with passion the mission of developing and spreading the discipline across the country and with various medical communities. The benefits of mesotherapy are twofold: doctors may easily learn the technique, while patients can have access to efficient and noninvasive medical technique. The nonsurgical aspect of mesotherapy makes it suitable for practice and potential insertion in the training curriculum of doctors hailing from the following specialties: sports medicine, rheumatology, dermatology, and for general practitioners too.

Here is to hope that one day, mesotherapy acquires the status and the fate it deserves in India.

Ajay Rana

ACKNOWLEDGMENTS

We would like to thank Dr Denis Laurens, President of the French Society for Mesotherapy, for write a Foreword and for having so warmly supported our project.

We want to express our sincere appreciation to our family, for helping us in the run-up to this book.

Finally, it gives us great pleasure to thank Shri Jitendar P Vij (Group Chairman), Mr Ankit Vij (Managing Director) and Mr MS Mani (Group President) of M/s Jaypee Brothers Medical Publishers (P) Ltd, New Delhi, India, for publishing our work.

CONTENTS

1. History of Mesotherapy 1
2. Mesotherapy Equipment 8
3. Medicines Used in Mesotherapy 13
4. The Rebound Effect 15
5. Cautions 16
6. Therapeutic Strategy 18
7. Techniques of Injections in Mesotherapy 19
8. The Mesotherapy Consultation 27
9. The Side Effects of Mesotherapy 28
10. The Pain Management 70
11. Mesotherapy Applications in Aesthetic 75
12. Alopecia and Mesotherapy (Hair Loss) 79
13. Cellulite: Mesotherapy Treatment 84
14. Vascular Pathology and Mesotherapy 87
15. Dermatologic Pathology and Mesotherapy 89
16. Mesolift 95
17. Scars 99
18. Keloid 101
19. Stretch Marks 102

Conclusion *105*

Bibliography *107*

Index *109*

1

HISTORY OF MESOTHERAPY

Dr Pistor was the inventor of *mesotherapy*.

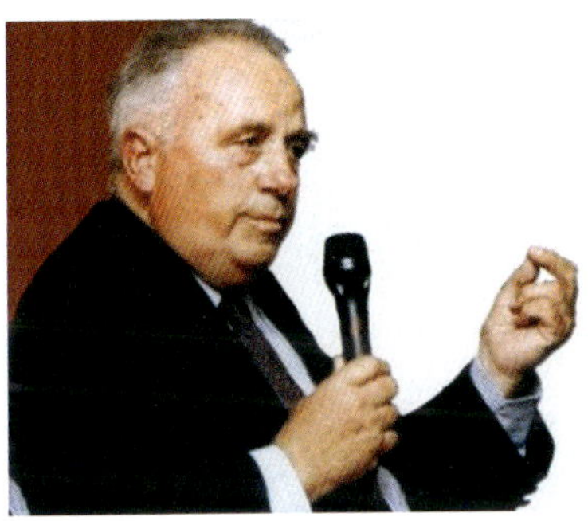

Dr Pistor began to practice in 1958 and discovered the interest of injecting small amounts of medications on the skin, first for pain relief, and had a particular interest for other applications like fat problems, cellulite, alopecia, venous insufficiency, and aesthetic and dermatological problems.

He used procaine for many purposes, which has since been replaced by xylocaine, lidocaine, and mesocaine.

Etymology of the Term Mesotherapy

Mesotherapy comes from—The Greek *mesos*, "middle" and therapy from the Greek *therapeia,* "to treat medically".

It means therapy within the mesoderm.

Originally mesoderm refers to one of the three primary germ cell layers in the very early embryo. It is not the real meaning of mesotherapy target.

So, many significations have been used.

Chronology

- Dr Pistor founded the *French Society of Mesotherapy* in 1964.
- The first *National Congress* occurred in 1976.
- Creation of the *Center of Research in Mesotherapy (CERM)* in 1981.
- Creation of the *International Society of Mesotherapy* in 1984.
- Recognition by the *French Academy of Medicine* in 1987.

Mesotherapy: An Interesting Alternative to More Traditional Therapies

Mesotherapy provides an interesting *alternative* to traditional therapies.

It is a *noninvasive* technique that patients appreciate, as it is painless and efficient. Another advantage is that the *cost* of the treatment is relatively low.

Fundamental Studies in Mesotherapy

Study Le Coz—Knee Articulation
Study—Dr Pitzurra/Questel
Double Blind Study—Le Coz/KacOhana
Pharmacokinetic Studies
Mixtures Compatibility Studies

Other Studies in Mesotherapy

Bibliographies of 1200 titles
Enatome I
Enatome II
Lumbago—Perrin
Lumbago. Art post—Ms/Infiltration—Mrejen
Pubalgia—Laurens/Demarais

Some Definitions to Begin

"The most allopathic of soft medicine and the most soft of allopathic medicine"
—Dr Pistor

Mesotherapy, "a royal way of introducing medicines", is an original technique of injection of micro-measured allopathic medicines, with a needle with cone Luer from 04 mm to 13 mm depth.

We owe this technique to Doctor Pistor, French doctor, who finalized the protocols of treatment of a large number of affections usually met in daily practice.

The injections are made, either in the hand, or with electronic devices of type Den' Hub" or "Pistormatic", or more rarely with devices of "mésoperfusion".

Used medicines are well-known and listed in the French pharmacopeia dictionary, and although the list of the available products is reduced, it is

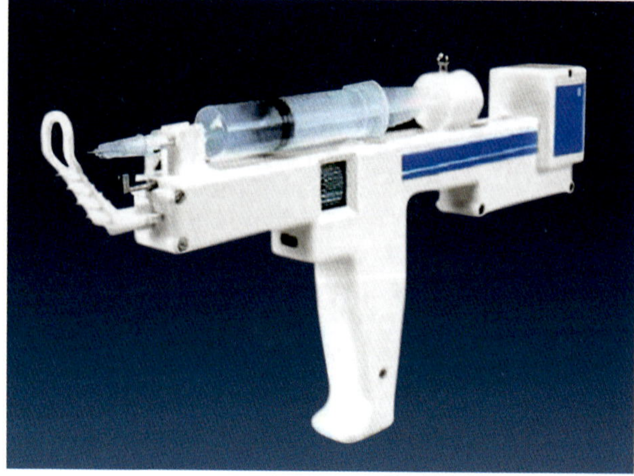

Fig. 1: Mesogun—Den' Hub.

possible to treat many pathologies, whether these are in rheumatology, in infectious, vascular pathology, etc.

The basic medicine of the mesotherapy was for a long time the procaine with acid pH, because of its fundamental properties, because it is thanks to it that are made (Fig. 1):

- The penetration of medicines which are associated to it
- The delayed effect which it confers on these medicines
- An effect of stimulation of the microcirculation
- An effect of immunizing stimulation:
  - An effect of regulation of the neurovegetative nervous system.
  - Procaine is always used, but, because of risks of allergy connected to its chemical composition, we prefer the xylocaine or the mesocaine.

No more than three products should be used in the same mixture, because after three medications one does not know what is working. However, one can make two separate mixtures in two different syringes.

The sessions are not too frequent in time: D0–D7–D14–D30 and every month or 2 months. It depends on the acute or chronic character of the pathology.

Why and How?

Innocuity or rare side effects—the medications we use are generally not dangerous if properly dosed. Some medications cannot be used together, for example calcitonin + anti-inflammatory, which makes a precipitate.

Some medications are contraindicated—no corticoids and risk of necrosis. No B_{12} vitamin in case of cancer story, we shall develop it in the pharmacology subject.

Economy for the Health System

Because of the small amount of medications, patients do not have to use too much oral medications; it allows patients to decrease their consumption of drugs.

It explains the few number of sessions.

After a Precise Diagnosis

(We shall develop that in the consultation of mesotherapy), you can define the right mixture, the right number of sessions.

This is an etiopathogenic therapy corresponding with the pathology.

Mesotherapy uses the classic injectable medications, so it is easy to find them in the classic pharmaceutics centers.

Few Rarely On The Right Place (Dr Pistor)

How?

How does it works? (Supposed action)

There are several mechanisms involved in the act of mesotherapy:

- The action of the needle

- A pharmacological action of the medications
- A vascular action
- An immunologic action
- A neuroendocrine action
- Sometimes a placebo effect can occur.

Proper action of the needle: The simple action of the needle causes a vascular effect on the skin—vasodilatation and an action on the neurologic *gate control system*, which is blocking the pain receptors and promoting the endorphin secretion.

Endorphins are released by the ends of the descending nerve fibers or going down fibers that come down the spinal cord from the brain.

When we feel a certain level of pain, the descending nerve fibers release endorphins at the level of the spinal cord, where they meet the sensory nerves carrying the pain messages from our body.

This local release of endorphins by the nerve inhibits some of all the pain messages going up from the brain.

Skin Structure

It is important to recall the structure of the skin (Fig. 2) because it is the main place we have to work with.

The deeper you inject, the more you have risks of side effects, from a simple allergy to an anaphylactic shock.

It is necessary to have a resuscitation structure with oxygen and adrenalin (Fig. 3).

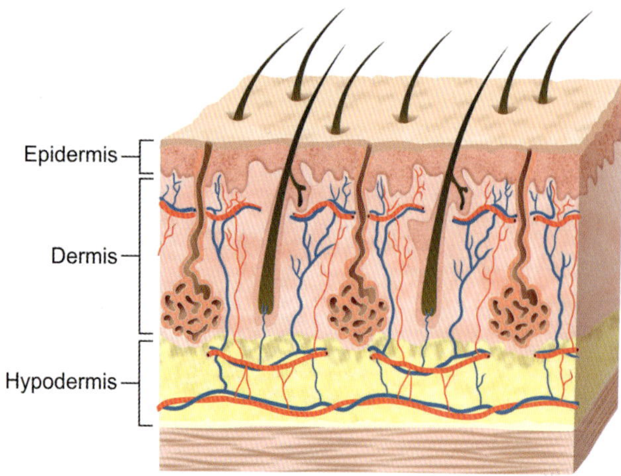

Fig. 2: Skin structure.

Theory of the four units of competence:

The structure of the skin depends of those four units:

1. Fundamental unit (extracellular matrix)

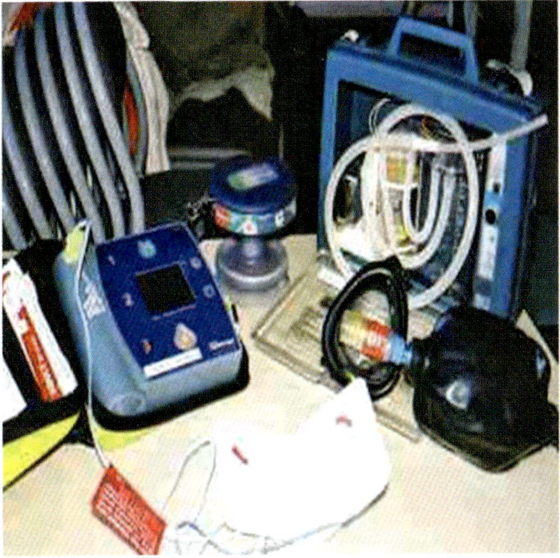

Fig. 3: Resuscitation material.

2. Circulation unit (arteriovenous system)
3. Neurologic unit: Sensitive nociceptive (afferent) and neurovegetative (efferent)
4. Immunitary unit.

Pharmacological Action of the Medications

Each medication has its specific action and must be properly adapted to the pathology.

The *pharmacology* studies:

- The action mechanism between an active principle and the organism in which it evolves, so it makes it possible to use those results for therapeutic purposes.
- The way to administrate the medications
- The side effects of those medications
- The medication interactions.

  There are the three notions to consider in the act of mesotherapy:

The pharmacopeia: It is a collection of regulatory official and authorized medicines in a country or a group of countries.

The pharmacodynamics: Studies the action of medication on the organism, and especially the interaction between receptor and the active principle.

The active principle diffuses in the site of action of the organ, combines with:

- Membrane receptor
- Enzyme
- Other cellular structure

And occurs a response.
The effects wanted or the toxic effects mainly depend on the concentration of medication on the site of action.

The Pharmacokinetics: Studies what happens in the organism to the active principle which is contained in the medication.

Four phases can be described: *Absorption, distribution, metabolization, and elimination* of the active principle (Fig. 4).

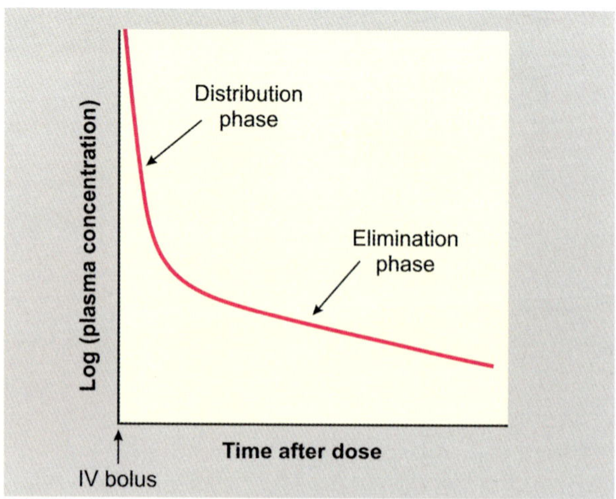

Fig. 4: Pharmacokinetics.

The Rules of Pharmacology in Mesotherapy

- *Primum non nocere*, which means—do not harm the patient
- One patient, one syringe, one needle, one bulb (ampule)
- Diluted, aqueous, and active
- Necessity of officially authorized medication
- Choice of the dilution product
- Choice of the associated product
- *Compatibility* between the products
- A *maximum of three products* in the mixture.

Vascular Action of the Mesotherapy

Important vasoactive effect with alternating vasoconstriction and vasodilatation (circulatory UC).

Immunologic Action

Pharmacological effect of the medications on the basal layer by immunostimulation (Fig. 5).

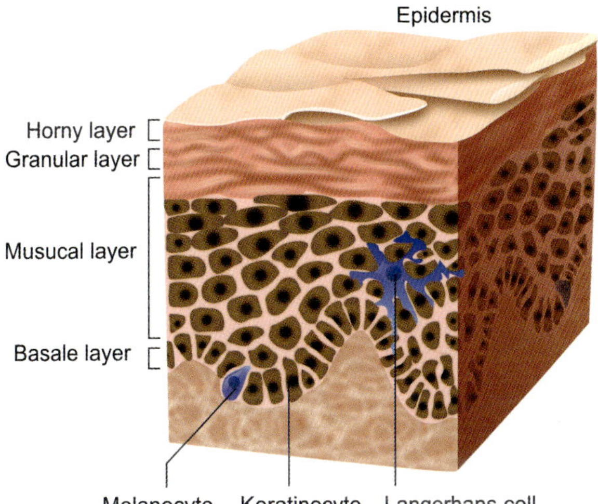

Fig. 5: Immunostimulation.

Neuroendocrine Action

Direct mechanical effect of the needle tip on the sensory receptors of the stratum corneum (Fig. 6).

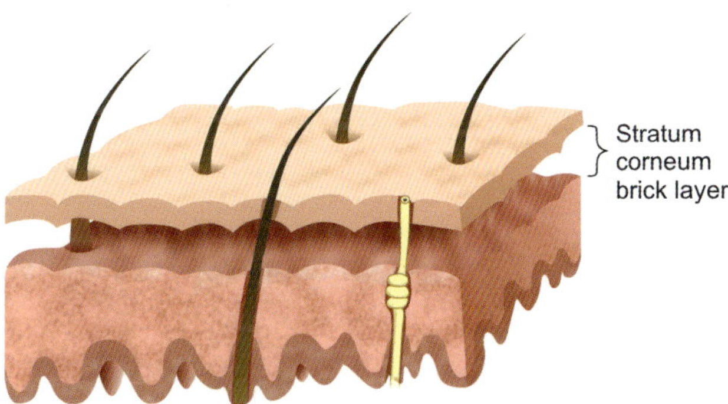

Fig. 6: Stratum corneum.

2

MESOTHERAPY EQUIPMENT

- The basic kit: Needle syringe (Fig. 7)

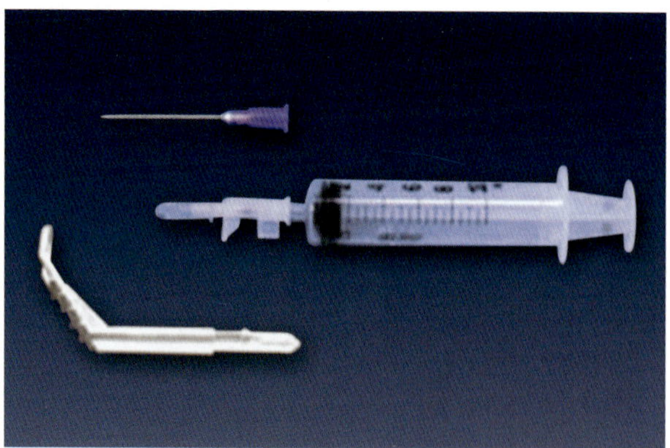

Fig. 7: The basic kit for mesotherapy.

- The types of needles (Fig. 8):
  - 32 G 0.27 × 13 mm: IED IDP DHD
  - 30 G 0.30 × 13 mm: IED IDS IDP DHD
  - 30 G 0.30 × 4 mm
  - 27 G 0.40 × 13 mm
  - 27 G 0.40 × 4 mm: IDS

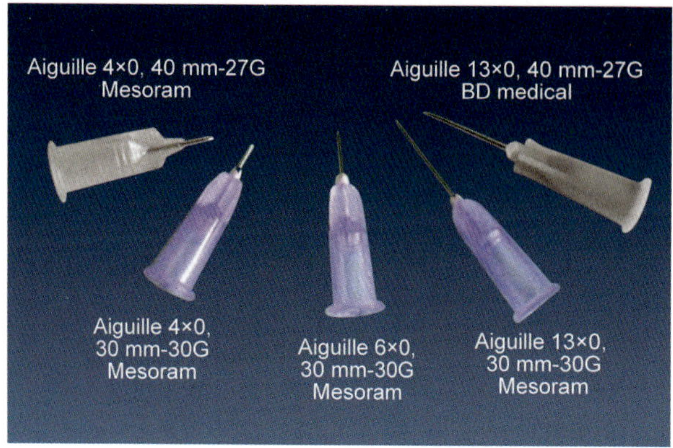

Fig. 8: Types of needles.

- The syringes:
  - Three sterile parts
  - Single use:
    - 1 mL
    - 2 and 2.5 mL
    - 5 mL
    - 10 mL
- The mesotherapy kits (Fig. 9):
  - Kit 10
  - Kit MPS
  - Mixt kit

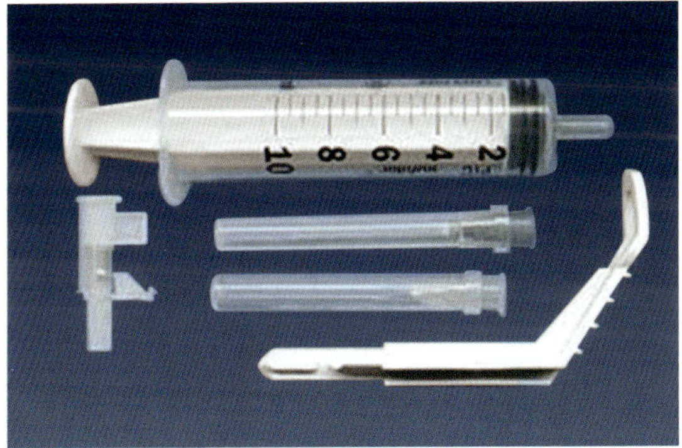

Fig. 9: Kit syringe + needle.

- The obsolete supports: Multi-injectors (Figs. 10A and B)

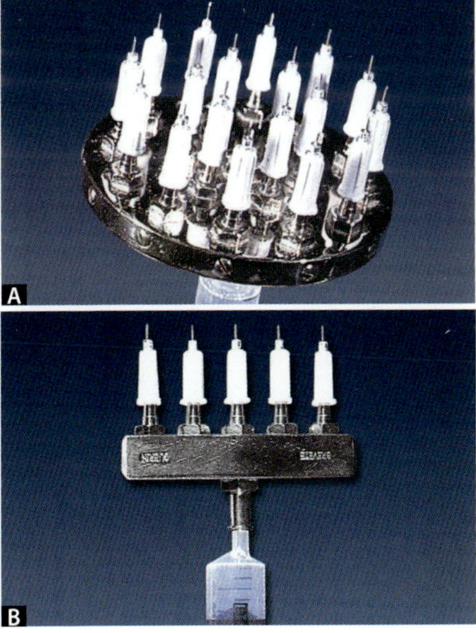

Figs. 10A and B: Obsolete supports.

- Forbidden material: The Mesoflash (Fig. 11)

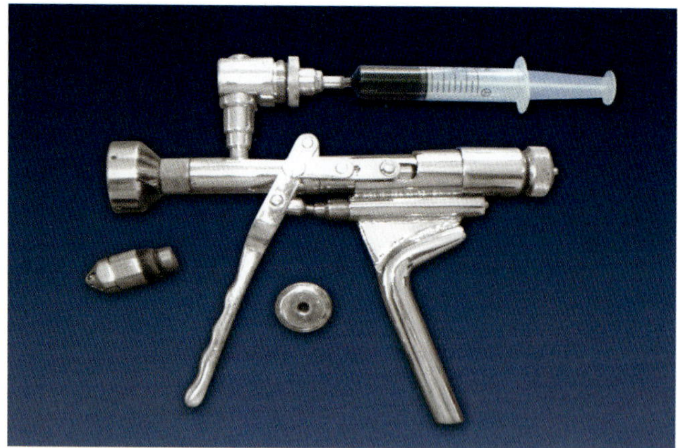

Fig. 11: Mesoflash—forbidden material.

- The different mesoguns (Figs. 12A to D):
  - The Den-Hub: DHN1, DHN2, DHN3, DHN4
  - The Pistor 1 and 2

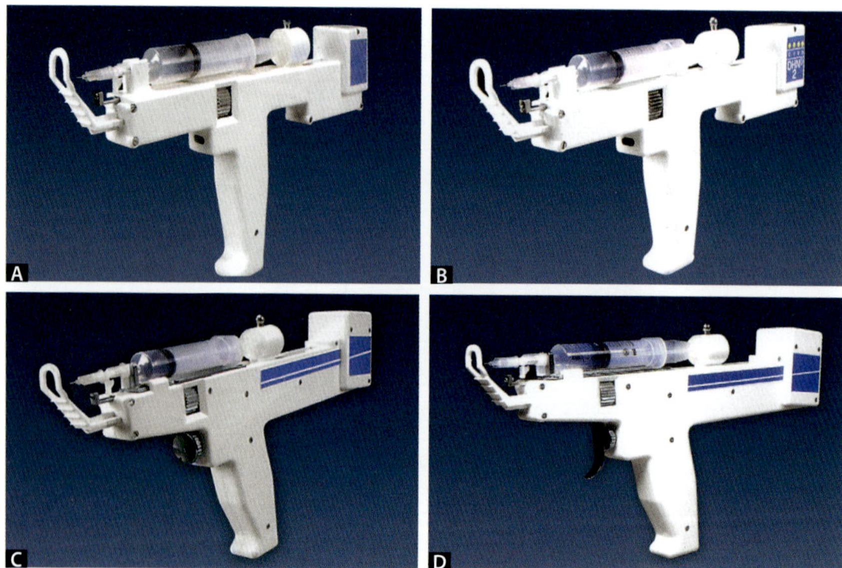

Figs. 12A to D: Mesoguns.

- The U 225 (Fig. 13)

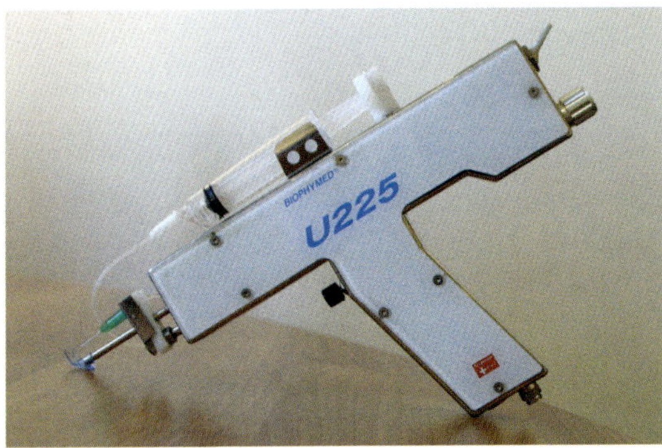

Fig. 13: U 225.

- The Mesalyse (Fig. 14).

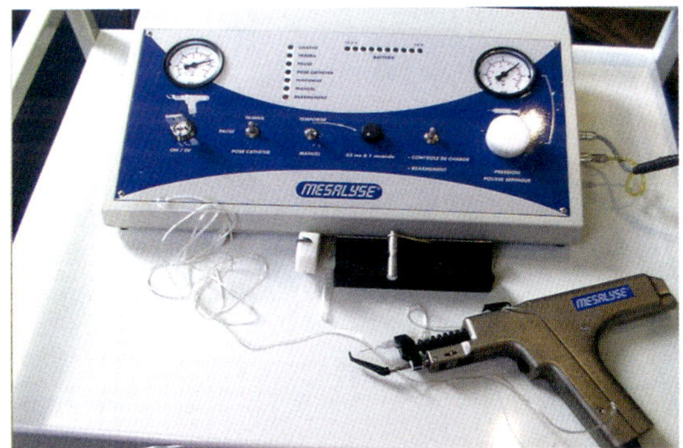

Fig. 14: Mesalyse.

After use, the needles must be put in special boxes for incineration (Fig. 15).

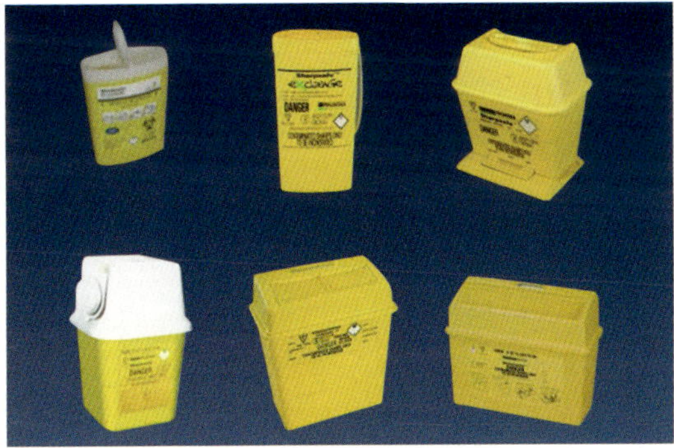

Fig. 15: Boxes for needle destruction.

Strict rules of asepsis must be applied, and the pistol and accessories have to be disinfected after every session (Fig. 16).

Products for disinfection: Alcohol 70%, Dakin, and Biseptine.

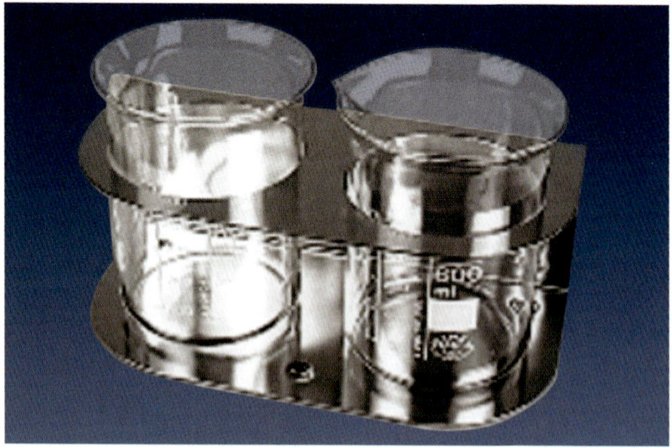

Fig. 16: Disinfection of the mesogun.

3

MEDICINES USED IN MESOTHERAPY

Allopathic Drugs

- Products for disinfection: Alcohol 70%, Dakin, and Biseptine (Fig. 17)
- Local anesthetics:
  - The procaine: Remained for a long time the "leader" of medicines used in mesotherapy; it is always of current use, but it is more and more replaced by the xylocaine, or the mesocaine (Rather in 0.5% dilutions).

    It is indispensable to ask patients about possible allergic reactions to local anesthetics!!!

    In the doubt, do not include these products to the mixture, and make your treatment with the other medicines used according to the pathology to be treated.
  - Diluting products: Physiologic serum and sterile water.
- Rheumatologic action: Calcitonin (salmon origin), myorelaxant (Thiocolchicoside), anti-inflammatories (piroxicam).
- Microcirculatory action: Etamsylate, terbutaline, arnica 4DH, propranolol (Migraine), and nootropyl
- Immunitary action: Anti-allergic polaramine
- Neurologic action: Laroxyl, rivotril, anafranil, and atarax
- Visceral action: Spasfon (phloroglucinol)
- Trophic and vitaminic action: Mag 2 (magnesium pidolate), vitamin C, vitamin B_6
- Thiamine (Vitamin B_1), Bepanthen, Biotin

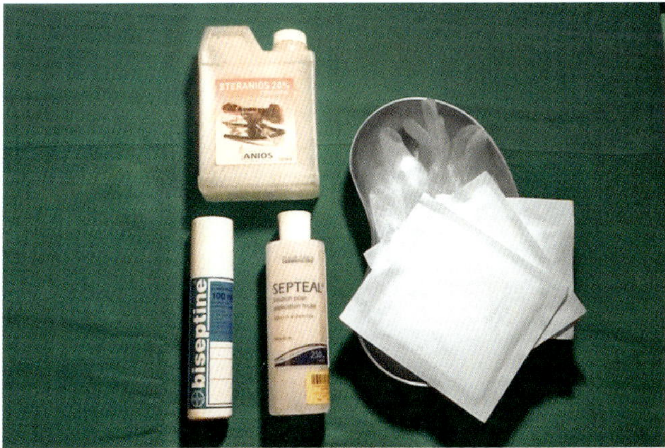

Fig. 17: Current disinfection.

- Vitamin B_{12} (not if story of cancer), organic silicium (degenerative pathology, cutaneous weakness)
- Vitamin E is no more used in France: Possible anaphylactic reactions.

Homeopathic Drugs

For example: *Rutin, Hamamelis, and Melilot* in the treatment of venous insufficiency.

Arnica: 4DH, indicated in bruises caused by acute sprains, contusions from direct traumas. It can be injected in a pure compound form or in combination with other mixtures to reduce the onset and severity of bruises.

Forbidden Drugs

- Corticoids
- Local anesthetic with adrenalin
- Alcoholic products or oiled products
- No authorized injectable products
- Antibiotics
- Low molecular weight heparin
- Golden salts.

What can be Treated in Mesotherapy?

- Pain
- Rheumatology: Arthrosis, osteoporosis, algodystrophy (complex regional pain syndrome)
- Traumatology: Sport injuries, tendinitis, epicondylitis, sprain, back pain
- Post-surgery
- Migraine.

Dermatologic and Aesthetic Applications

Mesorejuvenation, mesotherapy for fat and cellulite, wrinkles, and scars.

Other Indications

- Allergy
- Infectious diseases no more treated
- Vascular pathologies: Arteritis, venous insufficiency
- Anxiety and nervous breakdown.

4

THE REBOUND EFFECT

Something you should be aware of:

- There might be, the day after the session, a rebound effect, especially in the treatment of chronic pathologies for which vasoactive medication is used.
- This means that there will be a small rebound effect of the pain for the patient.
- This may last up to 24 hours and is nothing to worry about.
- You should warn the patient about this possible side effect.

CAUTIONS

- Do not harm the patient!
- One patient, one syringe, one needle
- Allergy
- Pregnancy and lactation
- Rigorous asepsy, double disinfection, and gloves
- No more than three products in one syringe
- Correlation between physiopathology and the choice of the mixture
- Dilution of the anti-inflammatories.

Other Cautions (Figs. 18 and 19)

- Patient with antithrombotic treatment, it is not a contraindication, but you have to control coagulation tests.
- As well, a patient with stomach ulcer can be treated with a few amount of anti-inflammatories, and you can complete with a protecting treatment like omeprazole.

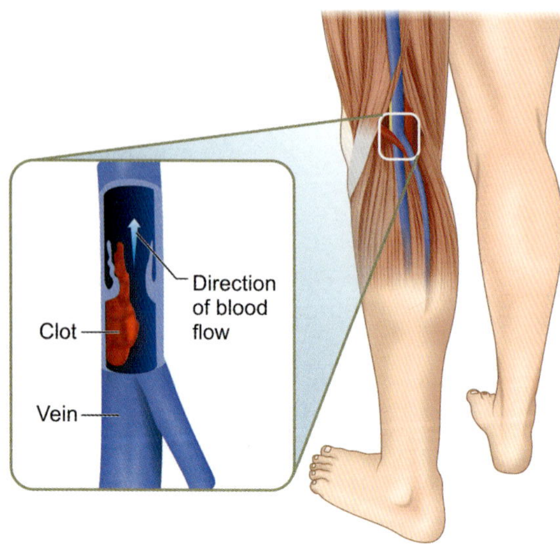

Fig. 18: Thrombophlebitis.

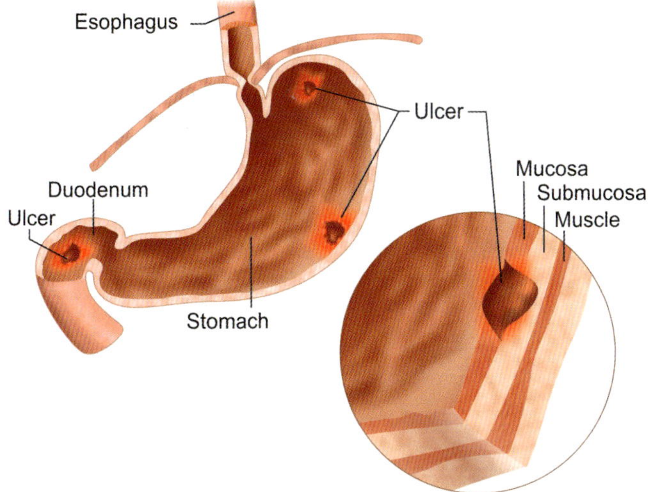

Fig. 19: Peptic ulcer disease.

6

THERAPEUTIC STRATEGY

We should ask ourselves some questions:

- *What tissue structure:* Synovial, tendon, ligament, muscle, nervous, and vascular
- *What story of the patient:* Age, pat pathologies, current treatment, duration of the most recent pathology, and skin quality
- *What painful points*
- *What rhythm for the sessions:* Acute or chronicle pathologies
- *What advices for the patient:* Life hygiene, quality of food, micronutrition, ergonomy (activity or rest)
- *What results you can anticipate for your patient*
- *What to do in case of failure:*
  - Rediscuss the diagnosis
  - Get a specialized advice.

TECHNIQUES OF INJECTIONS IN MESOTHERAPY

The classification of the techniques of injection is the result of a consensus with the Scientific Council of the SFM established in 1999.

The Objectives

- To know the skin structure and the different depths associated to the different techniques
- To know the interest of the different techniques and their applications (Fig. 20).

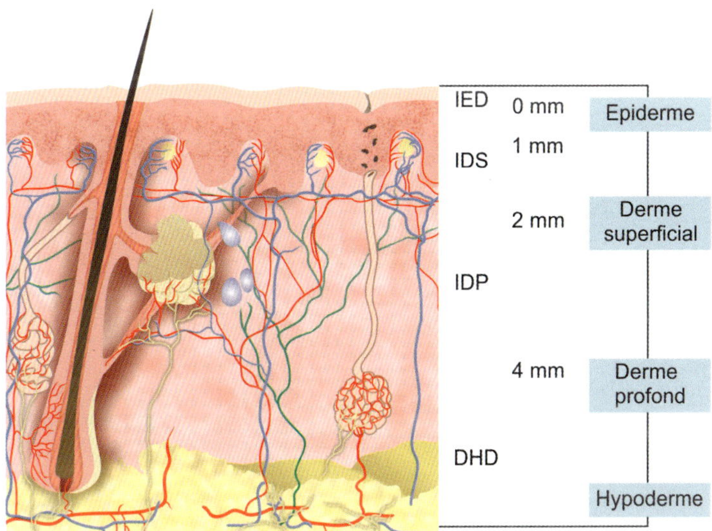

Fig. 20: Skin structure.

The Concept of the Four Unities

- Unity of *circulatory* competence
- Unity of *neurologic* competence
- Unity of *immunity* competence
- Unity of *fundamental* competence.

Notion of Mesotherapic Interface

Surface of contact between the mixture injected and the host tissues.

It will depend on the amount of puncture and the amount of activated skin receivers of the different unities of competence.

The multiplication of the punctures increases the mesotherapic interface.

Mesotherapy Techniques

- Intraepidermal
- Papular
- Nappage
- Point by point
- Mesoperfusion—obselete
- Punctilious systemized mesotherapy.

Intraepidermal

- Technique applied on to the epidermis
- Simple, painless, and no bleeding
- Allows usage of all medications
- Major stimulation of the skin
- Rapid onset of action
- Large surfaces covered
- All zones accessible.

Epidermic Mesotherapy (Perrin) (Fig. 21)

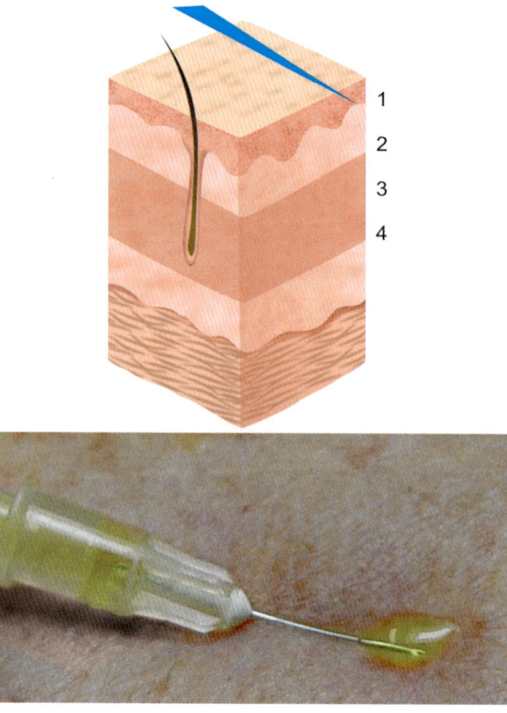

Fig. 21: Epidermic mesotherapy.

Intraepidermal (Figs. 22 and 23):

- A 13-mm needle (30G) is used for this injection technique.
- Needle *tangential* to the skin, *bevel up*, needle pointing always in contact with the skin.

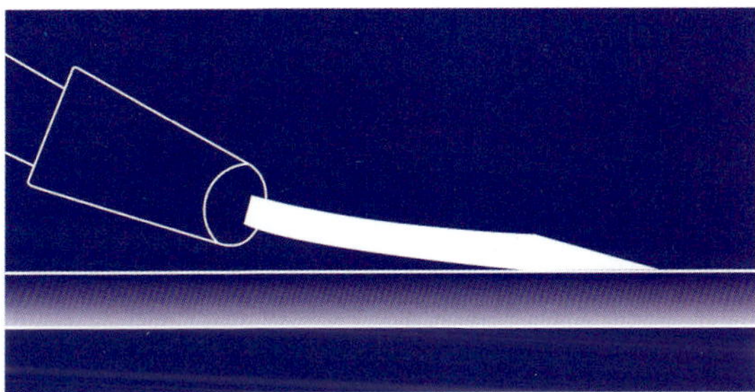

Fig. 22: Inclination of the needle.

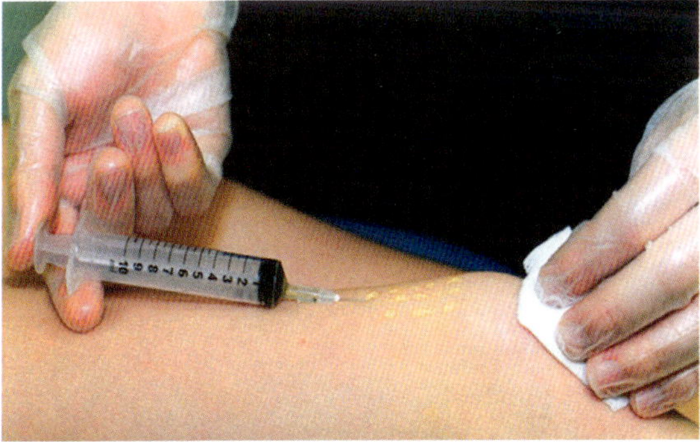

Fig. 23: Intraepidermal injection.

- Multiple small punctures on the epidermis at a depth not exceeding 1 mm are performed with quick synchronized flicking movements of the practitioner's wrist.
- The product is not injected into the skin but deposited on its surface by the multiple injections, allowing it to be quickly absorbed.
- It is very important not to clean the skin too soon, the medication should stay on the skin so as to allow a slow absorption of the medicine into the basal layer of skin. This slow absorption is the most important aspect of the technique.
- Beware skin abrasions and bleeding.
- Ideal for patients with *low pain threshold.*
- Ideal for *facial rejuvenation*—mesolift and mesoglow.

Pressure: 40 gramme; Angle: 15°

IDS (Nappage) (Fig. 24)

Advantages:

- Major stimulation of the skin
- Large surfaces covered
- Little pain (if done correctly)
- Rapid onset of action
- Ideal for scalp treatment
- Cellulite treatment for large surfaces like abdomen and back
- Technique can be applied with mesogun
- Ideal for fat reduction, cellulite treatment
- Little pain, pain usually when products are being delivered into the areas concerned.

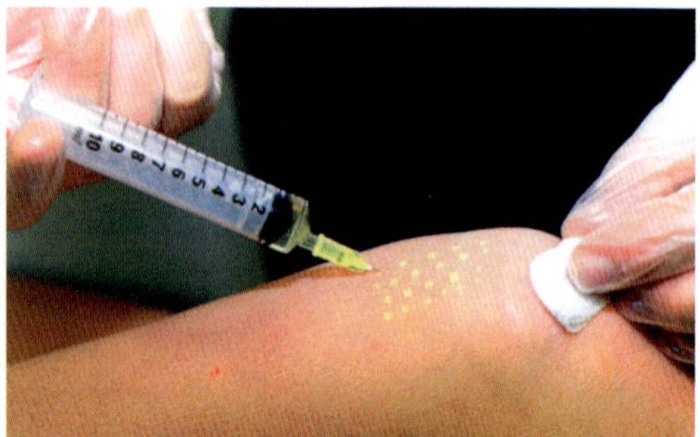

Fig. 24: Papular technique.

Papular Technique (Fig. 25)

- Tangential injection at the skin level, at the level of the basal layer, between epidermis and superficial dermis.
- Technique of injection applied to where epidermis meets dermis.
- Epidermis is actually lifted from the basal layer

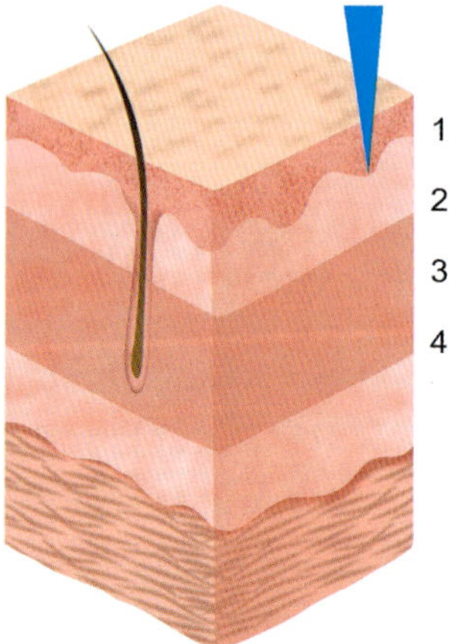

Fig. 25: Papular depth.

- Painful
- Ideal for treatment of wrinkles and scalp
- Hyaluronic acid rejuvenation.

Dry Mesotherapy (Fig. 26)

Superficial multipunctures at the level of epidermis and superficial dermis.

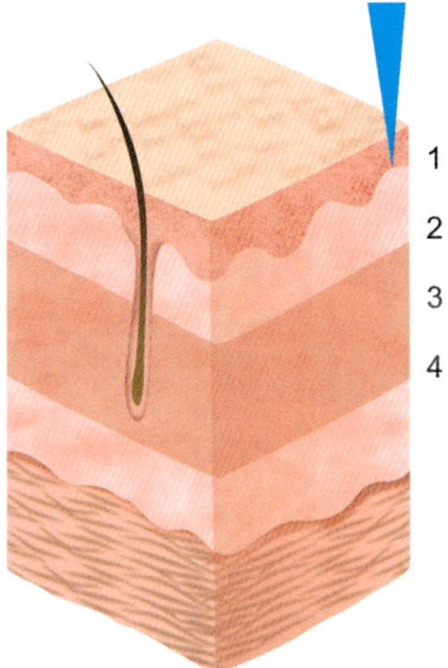

Fig. 26: Dry mesotherapy.

Point by Point (Fig. 27)

First described in the context of mesotherapy by Dr Pistor.

For point by point, we use a 4 mm or 6 mm needle which will be inserted perpendicularly to the skin to the hub.

It is also called IDP (In French: intradermique profonde)

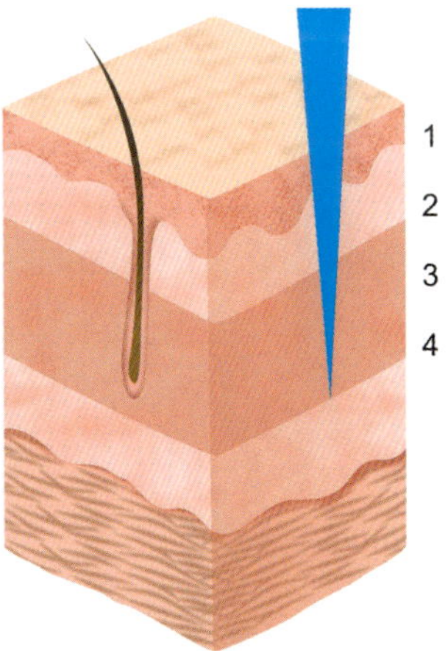

Fig. 27: Point by point depth.

We prick perpendicular to the skin, we inject, and we take out the needle (Figs. 28A and B).

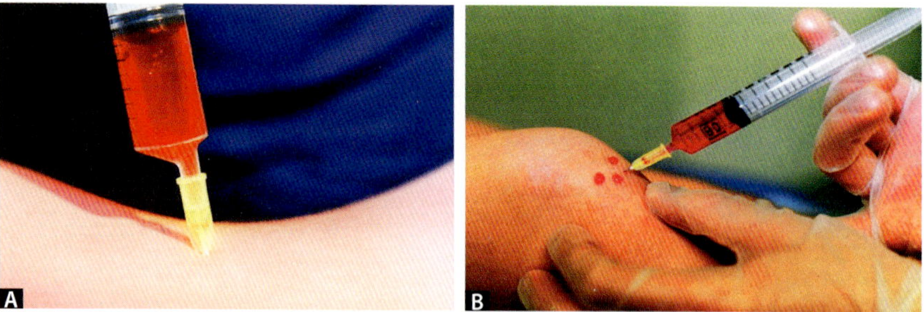

Figs. 28A and B: (A) Point by point; (B) Deep intradermic.

Slow Mesoperfusion (Fig. 29)

Technique of subcutaneous or intradermal injection between 2 mm and 13 mm, characterized by a short injection time followed by a long pause (sequential MP) or a very slow injection (continued MP).

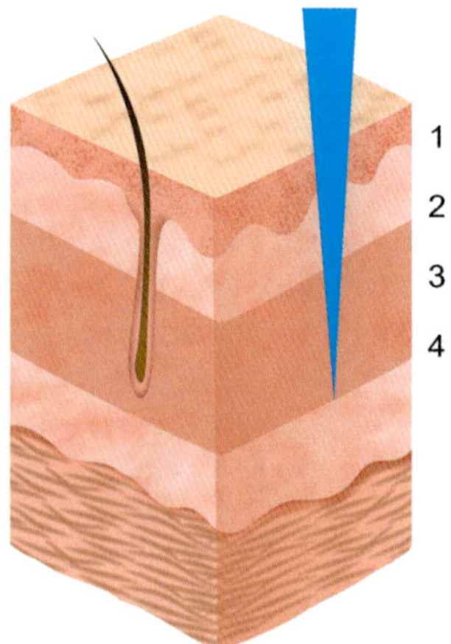

Fig. 29: Slow mesoperfusion depth.

Punctual Systematized Mesotherapy (Fig. 30)

MPS

- Hypodermic cutaneous injections
- On specific fixed points
- Those points are objective and reproducible
- They are necessary and sufficient.

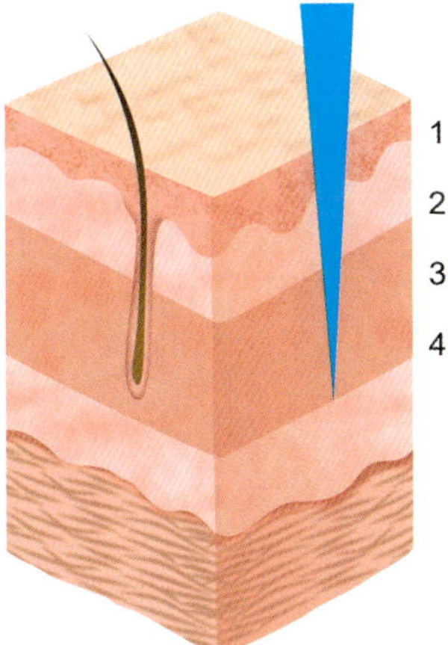

Fig. 30: MPS depth.

Let us resume the main techniques of injection (Figs. 31 and 32):

- The superficial techniques:
  - From 0 mm to 2 mm depth:
    - Epidermic mesotherapy (IED)
    - Nappage (IDS)
    - Dry mesotherapy
    - Papule
- Deep injections:
  - From 2.5 mm to 10 mm depth:
    - Point by point (IDP)
    - Mesoperfusion (MPL)
    - MPS (DHD).

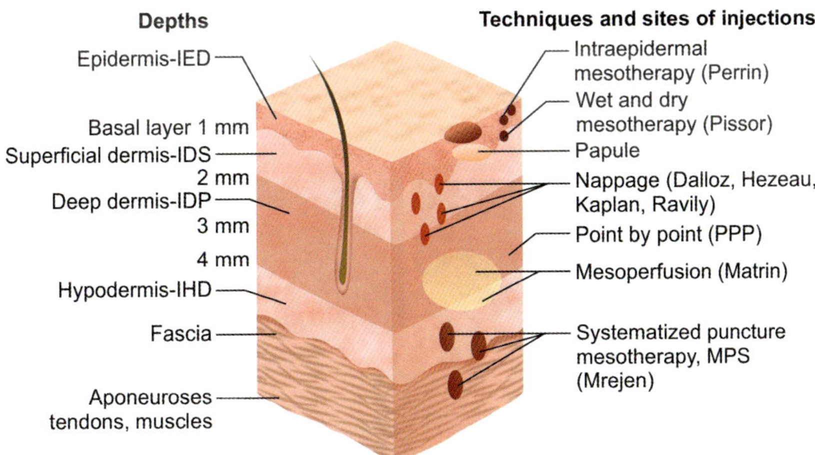

Fig. 31: Main techniques of injection.

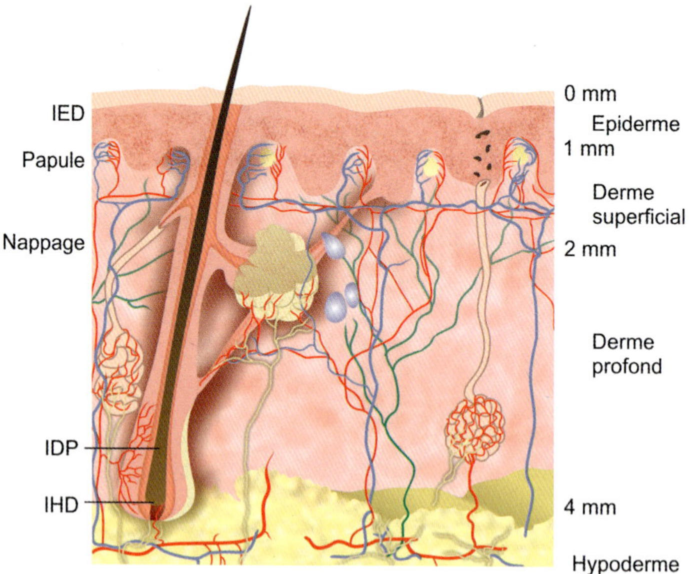

Fig. 32: The different depths of skin.

Summary: The Mostly Used Techniques ***(Figs. 33 and 34)***

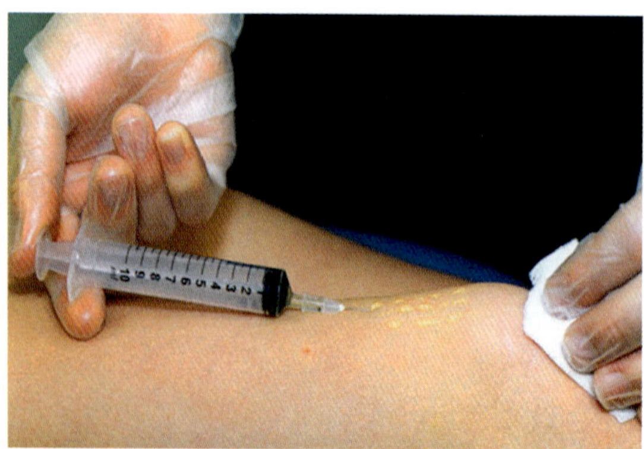

Fig. 33: Intra-epidermic technique.

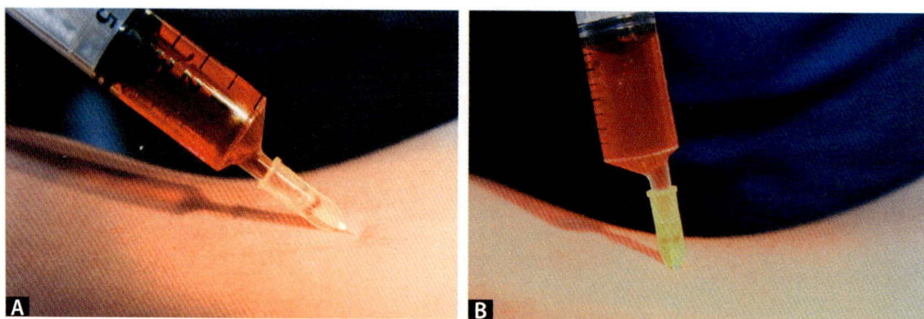

Figs. 34A and B: (A) Superficial intradermic (Nappage); (B) Deep intradermic (point by point).

8

THE MESOTHERAPY CONSULTATION

- Complete and precise clinic examination: Beware of allergies, immunity, diabetes, and infections
- Special precautions when:
    - Pregnancy
    - Menstruation
    - Fear of needles
    - Children under 12 years
    - Bad state: Diabetes and low immunity.
- How to treat: "Loco Dolenti", microdosed medication

Close to the area, no toxicity, efficiency, and long-lasting action.

THE SIDE EFFECTS OF MESOTHERAPY

Let us remind that it is necessary to have a resuscitation structure with oxygen and adrenalin.

The possible effects can be:
- Pain at the point of injection
- Bruises
- Allergy (type (chap) 1–3 or 4)
- Intolerance: Epigastralgia, flush, and lipothymic reaction
- Cutaneous necrosis
- Encysted bruises
- Rebound effect
- Mycobacteria infection.

Mycobacteria Infection (Fig. 35)

The main protocols used in mesotherapy:

It is important to notice that those protocols have been updated because some of the medications used in mesotherapy are less available in our country (For example: vasoactive drugs, immunostimulating drugs).

For some indications, it appears that some complementary techniques have a very interesting and synergic effect; we often use homeopathy, acupuncture, and auriculotherapy.

Moreover, it is fundamental, to insist on the thorough treatments, especially in the chronic pathologies, in particular in the treatment of arthrosis (anti-arthrosis medications, calcium, vitamins, oligotherapy, and homeopathy).

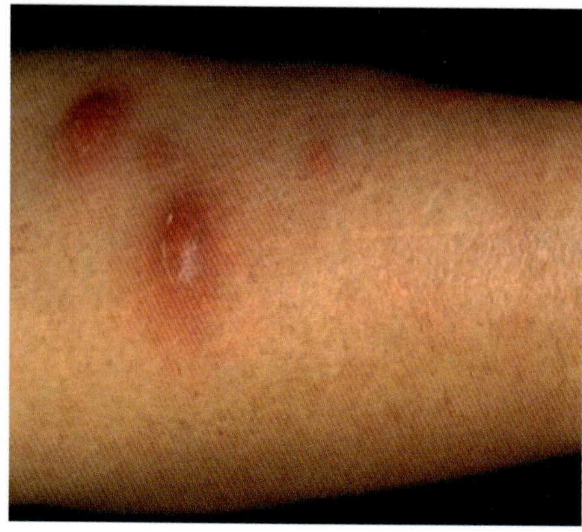

Fig. 35: Mycobacteria infection.

So, let us discover in the next pages what can be treated in mesotherapy.

You will have for every indication:

- The protocol
- The rhythm of the sessions
- The localizations for the injections

Technique of injection: When you see those symbols on the skin:

- --------------: Nappage
- xxxxxxxxx: Point by point
- 000000000: Deep injection (papular)

Acrosyndromes

These pathologies include:

- Acrocyanosis
- The Raynaud's disease
- Acroparesthesia

The origin is often genetic, and they occur mostly in cold seasons and in cold areas.

Protocol:

- Xylocaine 0.5%: 1 cc
- Etamsylate: 1 ampule
- Calcitonin 0.50 UI: 1 ampule

Rhythm of sessions: D1-D7-D15-D30 and once a month, in the cold period of weather.

Localizations (Figs. 36A and B): Along the affected areas: hands, or feet, arms, legs, and also along the lumbar zone chemical sympathectomy effect).

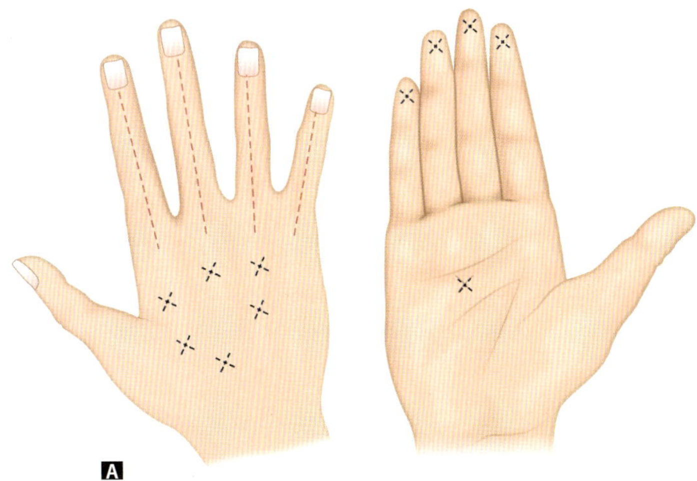

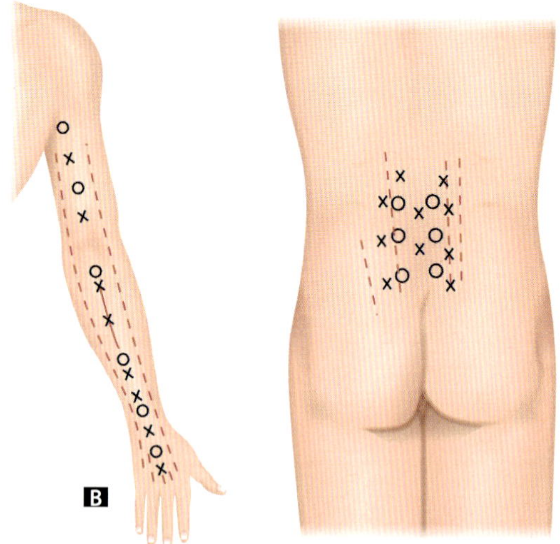

Figs. 36A and B: Acrosyndromes (Localization of injections).

Acrosyndromes (suite)

Technique of injection:

- --------------: Nappage
- xxxxxxxxx: Point by point
- 000000000: Deep injection (papular)

Aerogastria

This includes:

- Aerogastria
- Aerophagy
- Meteorism

It includes what we usually call *"Functional colopathy"*.

The protocol of colopathy can be coupled with the treatment of the neurovegetative dystonia (we shall talk about it in next chapters).

Protocol:

- Xylocaine 0.5% (1 cc)
- Phloroglucinol (2 cc)
- Magnesium (3 cc)

Rhythm of sessions: D1–D15–D30

Localization: Along the transverse, ascending, and descending colon and superficial injections on the abdominal area, with oblique lines making the shape of a Christmas tree (Fig. 37).

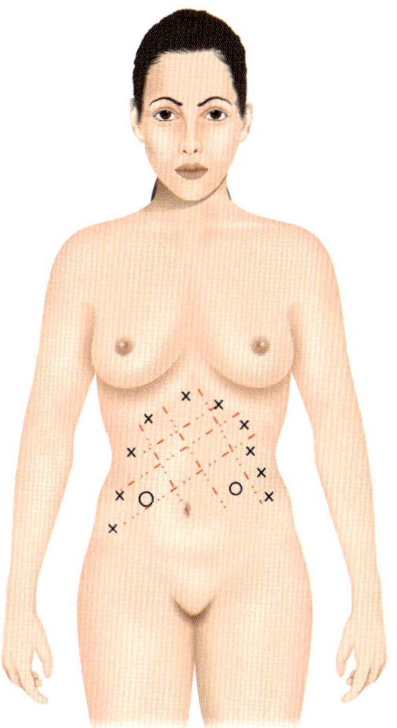

Fig. 37: Aecrogastria (Localization of injections).

Algodystrophy (Fig. 38)

A trivial complication in any joint surgery.

A syndrome featuring osteoporosis around joints, pain, swelling, excessive sweating, flushing and blanching of the skin and then atrophy, and loss of joint movement. It is probably due to disturbance of the sympathetic nervous system with interference with the small blood vessels. The condition usually clears up within a few months but there may be residual joint contractures.

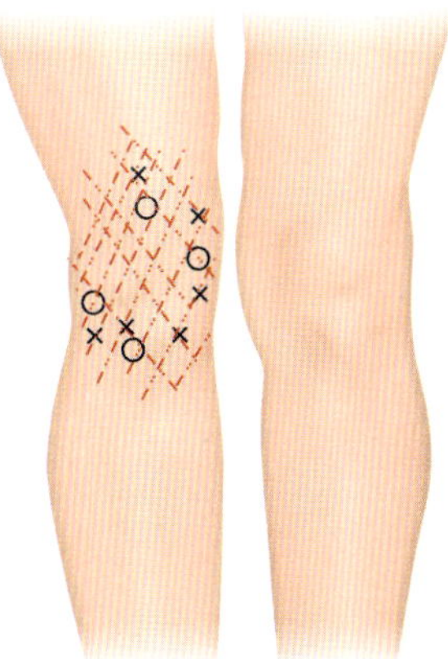

Fig. 38: Algodystrophy (Localization of injections).

Collins Dictionary of Medicine © Robert M Youngson 2004, 2005

The Protocol (Dr Laurens Denis, SFM PARIS):

Techniques: Mixt techniques: Point by point and intraepidermal

- Main mixture (point by point):
  - Terbutaline: 1 cc
  - Calcitonin 100 IU: 1 cc
  - Magnesium: 1 cc
- Complementary mixture (intraepidermal):
  - Xylocaine 05%: 1 cc
  - Thiocolchicoside: 2 cc

Application areas:

- The main mixture on the concerned articulation
- The complementary mixture on the periarticular area.

Rhythm of the sessions: D1–D8–D15–D30–D45–D60

Complementary treatment: Reeducation after D15

Allergy

See the chapters:

- Asthma (refers to page 36)
- Rhinitis (refers to page 63)

The basic protocol for all those indications is:

- Xylocaine 0.5% (1 cc)
- Polaramine: 1 ampule (antiallergic)
- Magnesium (1 to 3 cc, depending on the area)

Rhythm of the sessions: D1–D7–D15

Localizations: Depending of the pathology.
(See the chapters mentioned above)

Alopecia

This is a very interesting indication for mesotherapy, with good results on the feminine alopecia.
The male alopecia is more difficult to treat, the origin being different.

Protocol:

- Xylocaine 0.5%: 1cc
- Bepanthen: 1 ampule (Panthenol)
- Biotin: 1 ampule

Rhythm of the sessions: D1–D15–D30, and one session every month until the results are effective.

Localization: On the whole area of alopecia (Fig. 39).

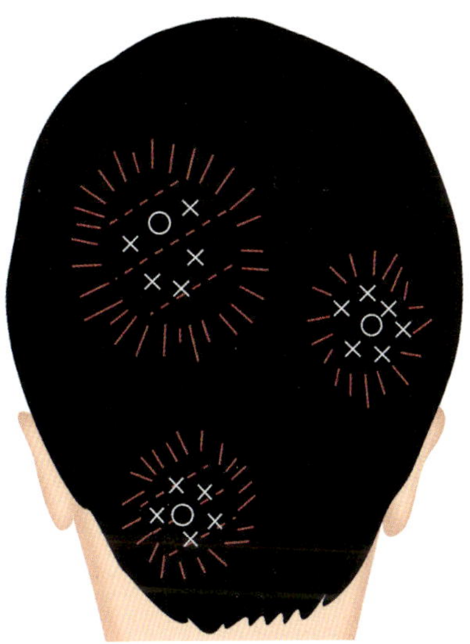

Fig. 39: Alopecia (Localization of injections).

Anxiety

Refer to the protocol of neurovegetative dystonia (NVD).

Arteritis (Lower Limbs Arteriopathy)

This is a very interesting indication and it is mostly recommended to treat this pathology as soon as possible.

"The sooner, the better", knowing that this pathology is evolutive and must be stopped before the necessity of the decision of surgery.

Protocol:

In France, we do not have pentoxifylline any more; we use etamsylate which is also a vasoactive drug.

So we use the following protocol:

- Xylocaine 0.5%: 1cc
- Etamsylate: 2 ampules
- Calcitonin: 1 ampule.

(The calcitonin has an anti-degenerating effect on the vascular system)

Rhythm of the sessions: D1–D7–D15, and then once a month.

Localization (Fig. 40): Along the lower limbs, and on the lumbar area (effect of chemical sympathectomy).

Arteritis (suite)

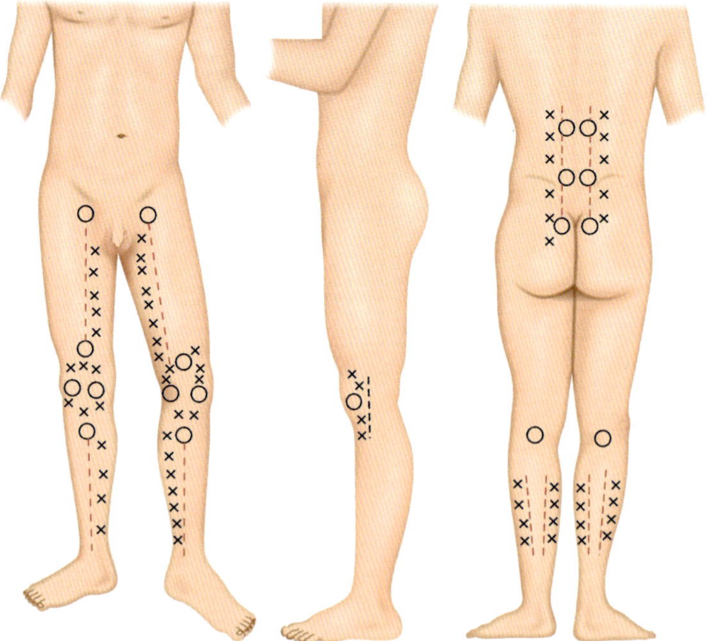

Fig. 40: Arteritis (Localization of injections).

Arthrosis

This is the most interesting indication in the practice of mesotherapy, and it takes the most important place in my consultations of mesotherapy.

There are two main protocols which can be used for those localizations:

- Arthrosis of cervical rachis
- Arthrosis of dorsal rachis
- Arthrosis of the lumbar and sacrum
- Arthrosis of the hips (coxarthrosis)
- Arthrosis of the knees (gonarthrosis).

The First Protocol (D1–D7)

It is used in the acute inflammation:
1st syringe:

- Xylocaine 0.5% (1 cc)
- Profenid (1 ampule)
- Magnesium (3 cc) for dilution.

2nd syringe:
Thiocolchicoside (1 amp) + Magnesium (2 cc)

The Second Protocol (D15–D30)

It is used for chronic period, in order to bring a better vascularization and a regeneration of the vertebral area.

1st syringe:

- Xylocaine 0.5%: 1 cc
- Etamsylate: 1 ampule
- Calcitonin: 1 ampule (for osteoporosis).

2nd syringe:

Magnesium: 2 cc + Thiocolchicoside (1 amp)

After the two protocols, you can make one session by month with the second protocol. It has a good effect on the general state of the patients, improves mobility, and make the pain decrease.

The localizations depend on the different pathologies.

Arthrosis (suite)

It is a good thing to associate different therapeutics:

- Anti-arthrosis medications
- Vitamins
- Oligotherapy
- Homeopathy-acupuncture
- Physiotherapy

Asthenia

We do not have any more medication initially used for this indication; nevertheless it is possible to use a mixture including vitamins, vasoactive drugs, and calcitonin.

It allows a better diffusion of the active medications by the way of microcirculation.

This microcirculation goes less and less effective as long as the patient gets older.

Protocol:

- Xylocaine (1 cc)
- Hydrosol polyvit (1 ampule)
- Etamsylate (1 ampule)
- Calcitonin (1 ampule).

It is interesting to associate medications like vitamins and oligotherapy.

The rhythm of sessions: D1-D15-D30.

Localization: All along the rachis (see the picture for neurovegetative dystonia, refers to page 53).

Asthma

Protocol:

It is the protocol used for allergy:

- Xylocaine 0.5% (1 cc)
- Polaramine: 1 ampule (antiallergic)
- Magnesium (3 cc).

Localizations

- All the area of the lungs (front, back, and sides) (Fig. 41)
- The Waldeyer immunocompetent zone (Fig. 42).

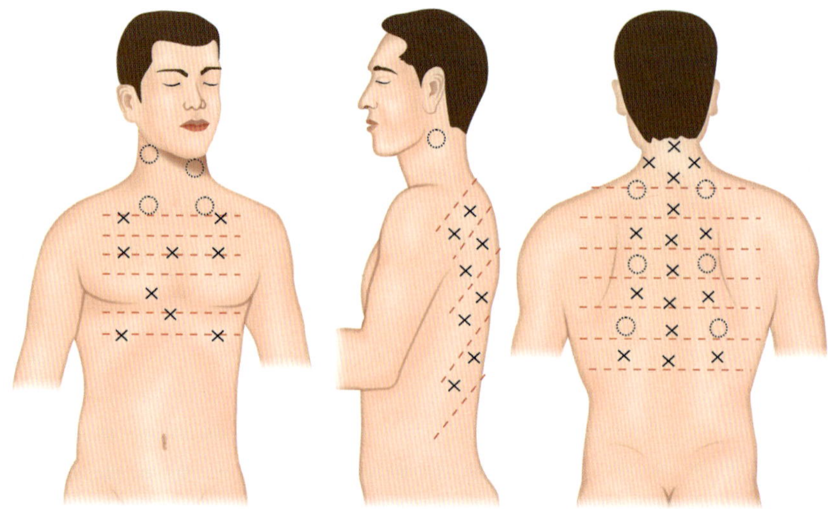

Fig. 41: Asthma (Localization of injections).

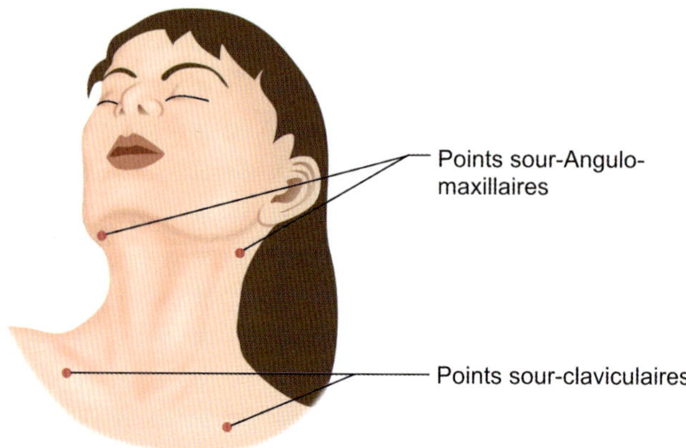

Fig. 42: The Waldeyer area.

Associated treatments:
- Antiallergic medications
- Inhaled corticoids and bronchodilators.

Acouphenes (Humming of Ears)

Protocol:
- Xylocaine 0.5% (1 cc)
- Etamsylate (1 ampule)
- Calcitonin (1 ampule).

Rhythm of the sessions: D1–D7–D15

The sessions can be proposed again in case of new episodes of humming.

Localizations (Fig. 43):
- Around the ears
- Along the carotids.

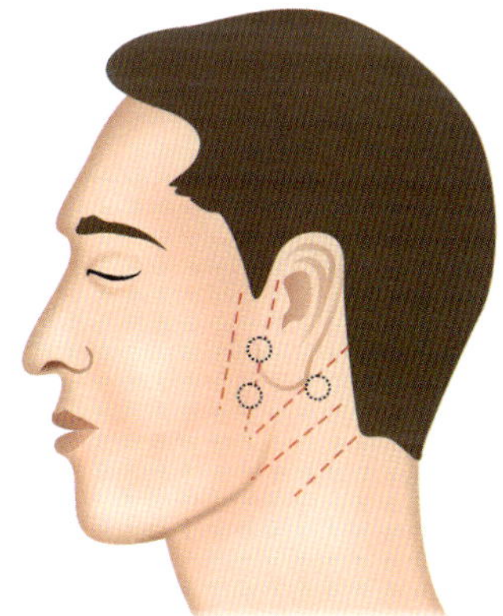

Fig. 43: Acouphenes (Localization of injections).

Cataract

In this indication, the purpose is to stop the lens degenerescence by bringing calcitonin and vasoactive medication (etamsylate).

We have to treat as soon as possible, before the vision is too much affected.

Protocol:
- Xylocaine 0.5% (1 cc)
- Etamsylate (1 ampule)
- Calcitonin (1 ampule).

Rhythm of the sessions: Every 2 or 3 months.

Localization: Around the eyebrows; one continuous injection each side (Fig. 44).

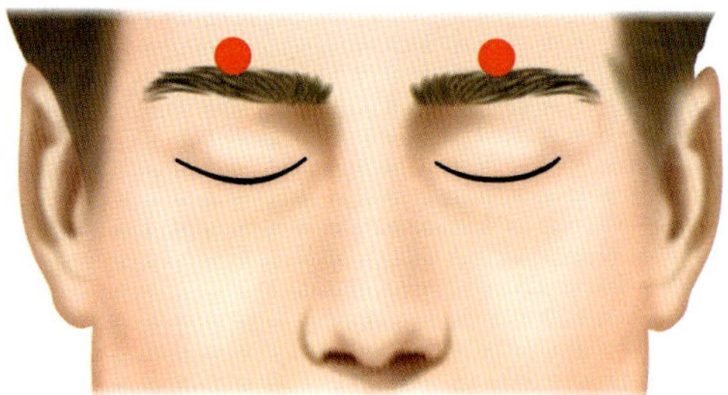

Fig. 44: Cataract (Localization of injections).

Cephalalgia (Headache)

Please refer to the chapters:
- Cervicodynia
- Cervical arthrosis
- Migraine (refers to page 52).

Cervicodynia (Headaches of Cervical Origin)

Protocol:
- Xylocaine 0.5% (1 cc)
- Thiocolchicoside (1 amp)
- Magnesium (3 cc).

Rhythm of sessions: D1–D7–D15.

Localization (Figs. 45A and B):
- Temporal zones

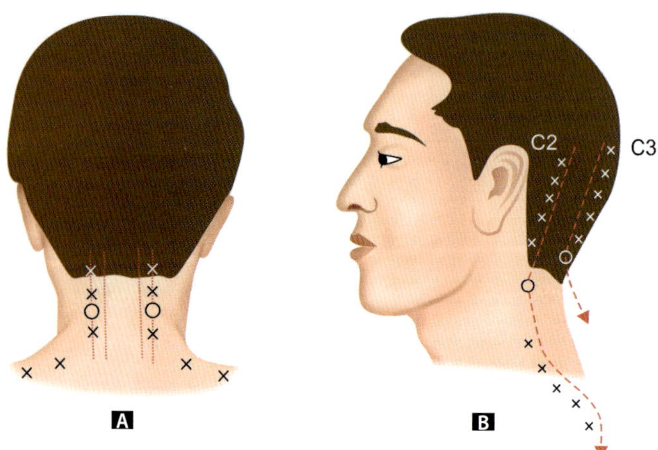

Figs. 45A and B: Cervicodynia (Localization of injections).

- Cervical spine
- Surrounding muscles.

Cervical Arthrosis

Protocol: The same as the one we use in arthrosis depending on the evolution—acute or chronical.

Rhythm:
- D1-D7 (acute arthrosis)
- D15-D30 (chronical pain)

Localization: The same as cervicodynia.

Coccydynia

- Pain that occurs in the coccygeal area
- It is necessary to find the cause of that pain:
  - Post-traumatic?
  - Arthrosis?

If post-traumatic pain:
Use this protocol:
- Xylocaine 0.5%: 1 cc
- Diclofenac: 1 amp
- Magnesium (3 cc).

If the pain is caused by arthrosis:
See the protocol of arthrosis.

Localization (Fig. 46)

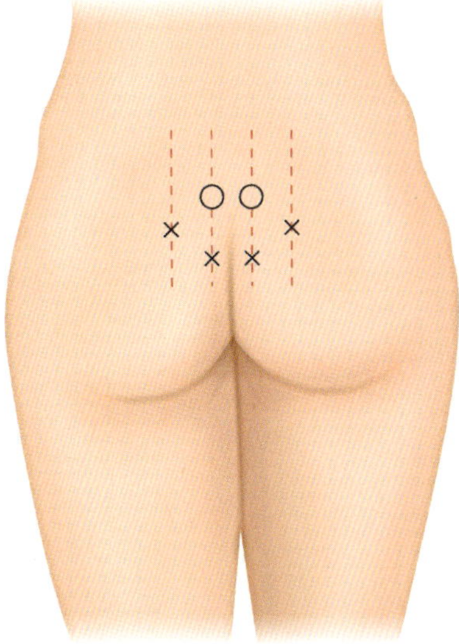

Fig. 46: Coccydynia (Localization of injections).

Colic: Hepatic Colic–Nephric Colic

Mesotherapy can help, completing the classic treatment of those pathologies.

Protocol:
- Xylocaine 0.5% (1 cc)
- Phloroglucinol (1 ampule).

Rhythm: When the crisis occurs.

Localization (Fig. 47)

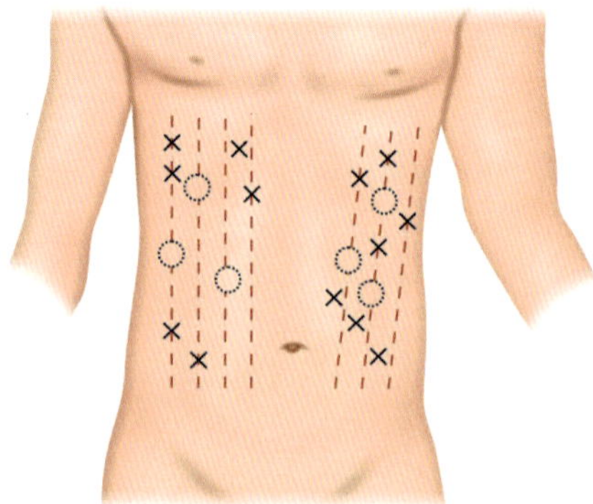

Fig. 47: Colic (Hepatic–Nephric) (Localization of injections).

Colopathy (and Constipation)

Protocol:
- Xylocaine 0.5% (1 cc)
- Phloroglucinol (1 ampule)
- Magnesium (3 cc).

This protocol can be combined to the treatment of NVD.

Rhythm of sessions: There is not a specific rhythm for this kind of pathology; you can treat every time the patient asks for a session.

It is important to combine hygieno-dietetic measures and a regular antispasmodic and probiotic treatment.

Localization (Fig. 48)

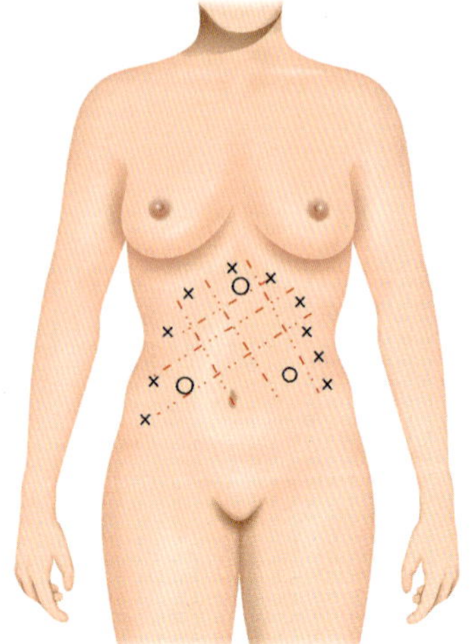

Fig. 48: Colopathy (Localization of injections).

Coxarthrose (Osteoarthritis of the Hips)

Protocol and rhythm of sessions: See the arthrosis protocol.

Localization (Fig. 49)

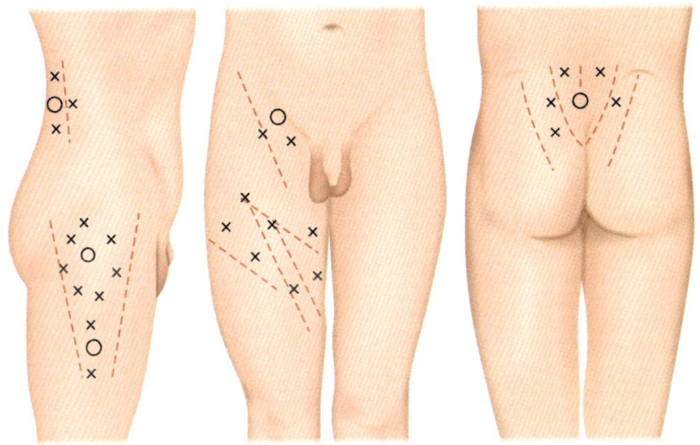

Fig. 49: Coxarthrosis (Localization of injections).

Cramp (Muscular Cramps)

First of all, it is essential to know the etiology of those cramps (metabolic, traumatic, and vascular).

Protocol:

- Xylocaine 0.5% (1 cc)
- Thiocolchicoside (1 ampule)
- Magnesium (3 cc)

It is possible to associate etamsylate (1 amp) when a vascular component is involved.

Rhythm of sessions: Every 3 months

Localization: On the area concerned, in this example, cramps in the leg (Fig. 50).

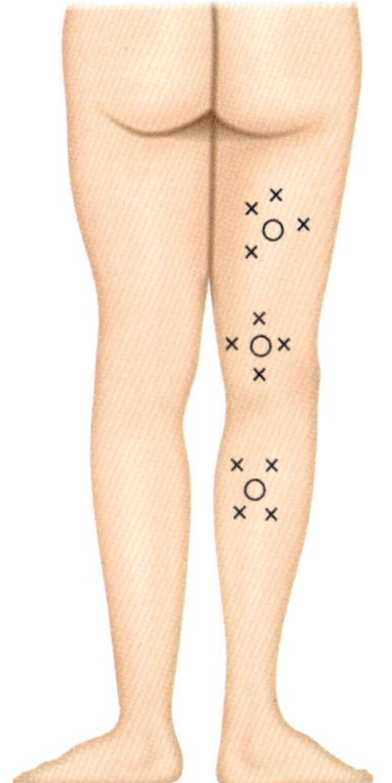

Fig. 50: Cramp (Localization of injections).

Depression (Nervous Breakdown)

Protocol:

- Xylocaine 0.5% (1 cc)
- Tofranil or anafranil (few drops)
- Mag 2 (3 cc).

Alternate with the NVD protocol:

- Xylocaine 0.5% (1 cc)
- Thiocolchicoside (1 ampule)
- Mag 2 (3 cc).

Localization: The same as the dystonia localizations (see the chapter NVD):

- Temporal zones
- Abdominal area
- Spinal cord.

Frequency of sessions: D1–D7–D15 and when needed.

Dysmenorrhea

Protocol:

- Xylocaine 0.5%: 1 cc
- Phloroglucinol: 1 ampule.

Alternate with the NVD protocol.

Localization (Fig. 51)

Frequency of sessions: Every 2 or 3 months.

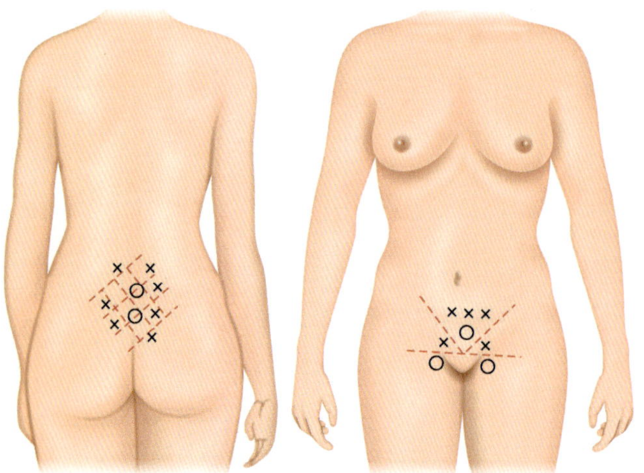

Fig. 51: Dysmenorrhea (Localization of injections).

Dyspepsia (Nausea)

Protocol:

- Xylocaine 0.5%: 1 cc
- Trimebutine: 1 ampule.

Alternate with the NVD protocol.

Localization (Fig. 52)

Frequency of sessions: D1–D7–D15 and when needed.

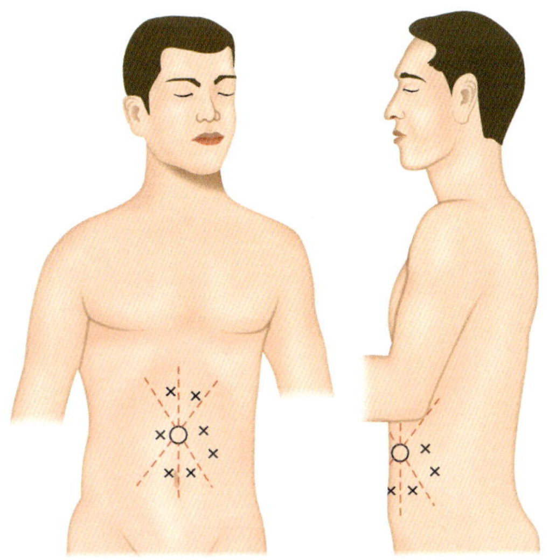

Fig. 52: Dyspepsia (Localization of injections).

Epicondylitis (Tennis Elbow)

Protocol:

- Acute period of inflammation:
  - Xylocaine 0.5%: 1 cc
  - Diclofenac: 1 ampule
  - Mag 2: 3 cc (dilution)
- Chronic period:
  - Xylocaine 0.5%: 1 cc
  - Etamsylate: 1 ampule
  - Calcitonin 50 UI: 1 ampule.

Localizations (Fig. 53)

Frequency of sessions: D1–D7–D15–D30.

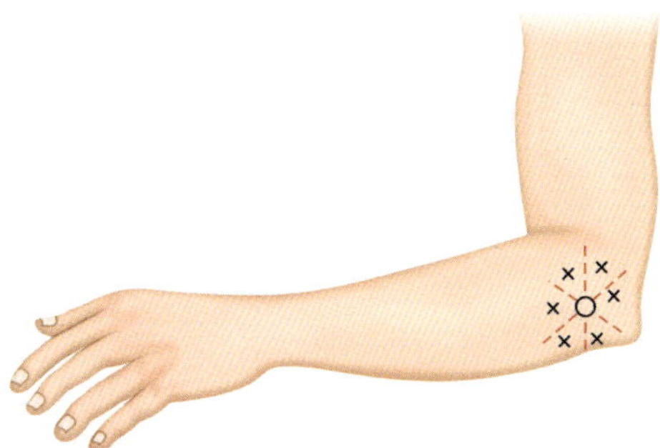

Fig. 53: Epicondylitis (Localization of injections).

Epiphysitis (Scheuermann Disease)

Protocol:
- Xylocaine 0.5%: 1 cc
- Calcium: 1 ampule
- Soluvit.

Alternate with NVD protocol.

Localization (Fig. 54)

Frequency of sessions: Every month.

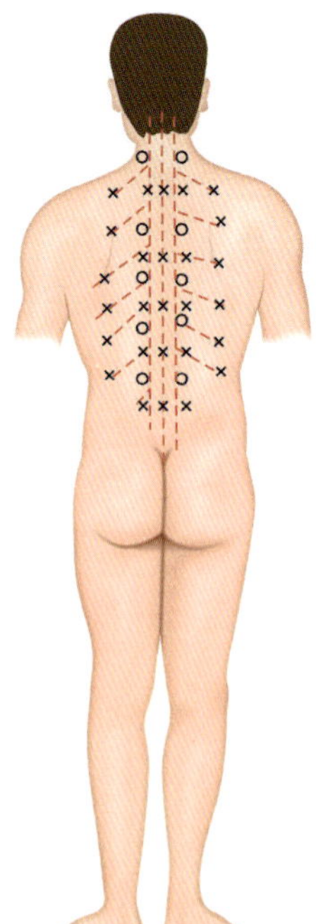

Fig. 54: Epiphysitis (Localization of injections).

Gastralgia

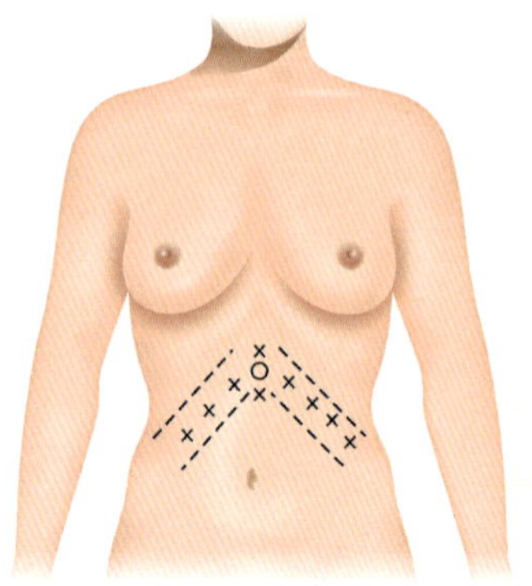

Fig. 55: Gastralgia (Localization of injections).

Protocol:
- Xylocaine 0.5%: 1 cc
- Trimebutine: 1 ampule.

Localization (Fig. 55)

Frequency of sessions: When needed.

(**Note**: It is important to make a precise diagnosis before the treatment, and appreciate if mesotherapy will be the right attitude for this pathology)

Hallux Valgus

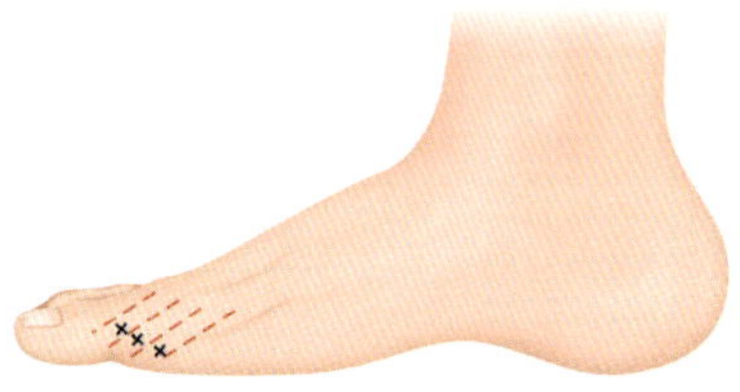

Fig. 56: Hallux valgus (Localization of injections).

Protocol: Same protocol as the arthrosis protocol.

- Acute period of inflammation:
  - Xylocaine 0.5%: 1 cc
  - Diclofenac: 1 ampule
  - Mag 2: 3 cc (dilution)
- Chronic period:
  - Xylocaine 0.5%: 1 cc
  - Etamsylate: 1 ampule
  - Calcitonin 50 UI: 1 ampule.

Localization (Fig. 56)

Frequency of sessions: D1–D7–D15, and then every month.

Hygroma (Elbow and Knee) (Figs. 57A and B)

Protocol:

- Xylocaine 0.5%: 1 cc
- Etamsylate: 1 ampule
- Calcitonin 50 UI: 1 ampule.

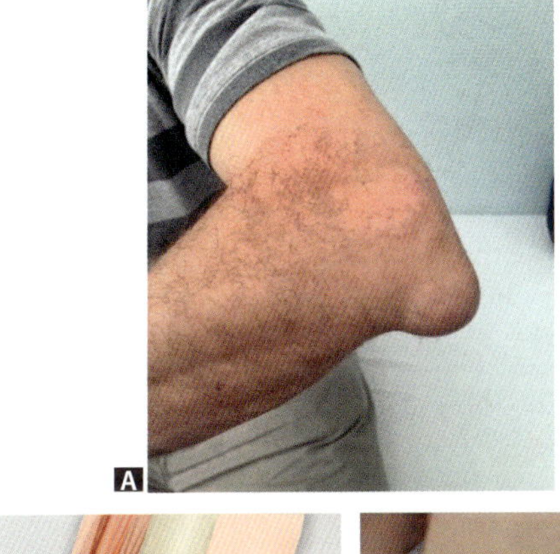

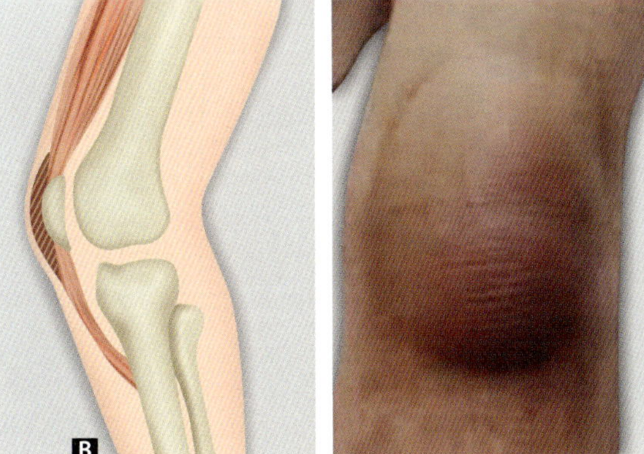

Figs. 57A and B: Hygroma (elbow and knee)

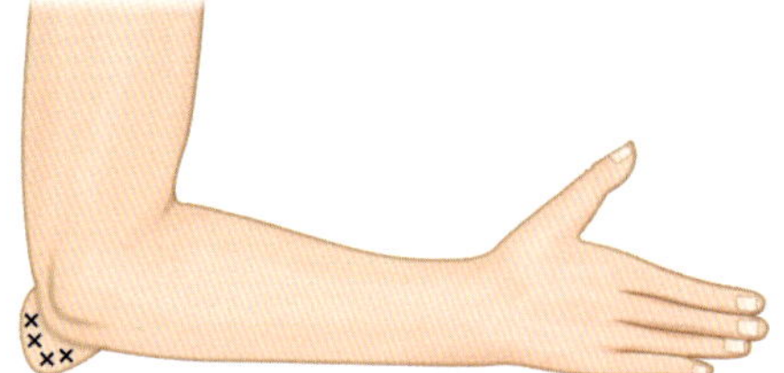

Fig. 58: Hygroma of the elbow.

Localization (here hygroma of the elbow, Fig. 58)

Frequency of sessions: D1–D7–D15.

Immunostimulation

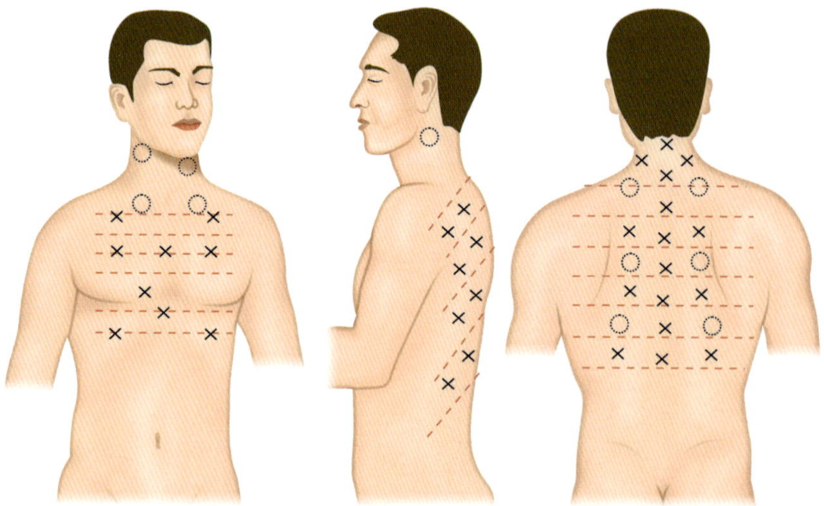

Fig. 59: Immunostimulation (Localization of injections).

The treatment of immunostimulation is a very interesting approach of the chronic infectious diseases; as we do not have any more the medications we used before in France, we can proceed with *"dry puncture"*.

The punctures can be applied on the areas of immunitary competence which can be seen in Figure 59.

Treatment on the lungs area projection:
This technique is very useful in chronic pulmonary diseases like chronic bronchitis, asthma, and sensitivity to infectious diseases.

The Waldeyer's ring area (Fig. 60):
Treating those areas improves the resistance to chronic pathologies of ORL pathologies: rhinitis, sinusitis, angina, amygdalitis.

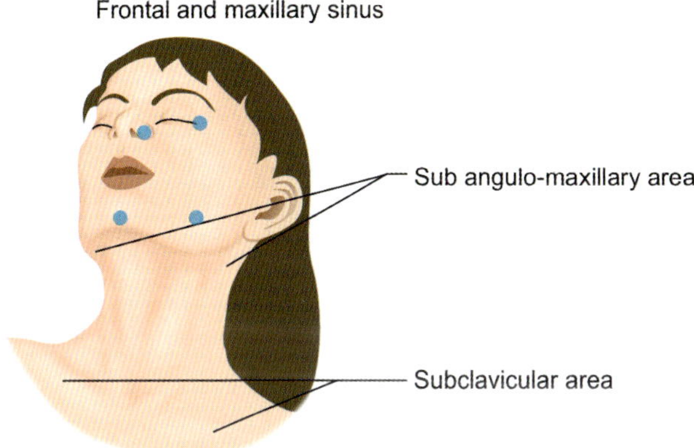

Fig. 60: Immunostimulation areas.

Dry Mesotherapy (Fig. 61)

Superficial multipunctures at the level of epidermis and superficial dermis.

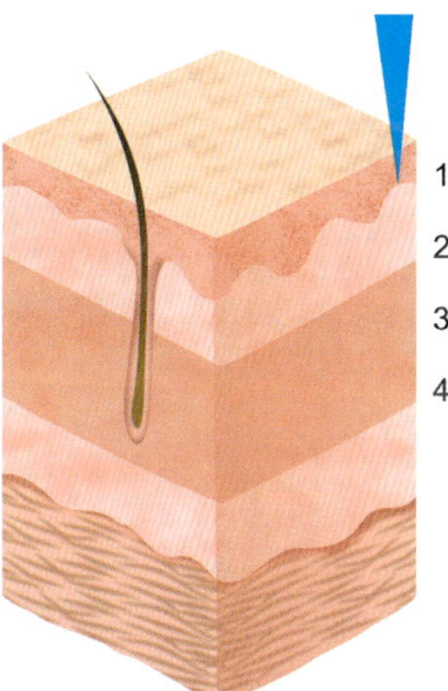

Fig. 61: Dry mesotherapy.

Insomnia

Protocol: The protocol is the same as the NVD protocol.

- Xylocaine 0.5%: 1 cc
- Thiocolchicoside: 1 ampule
- Mag 2: 1 ampule

Localization (Fig. 62)

Frequency of sessions: D1–D7–D30, and then when needed.

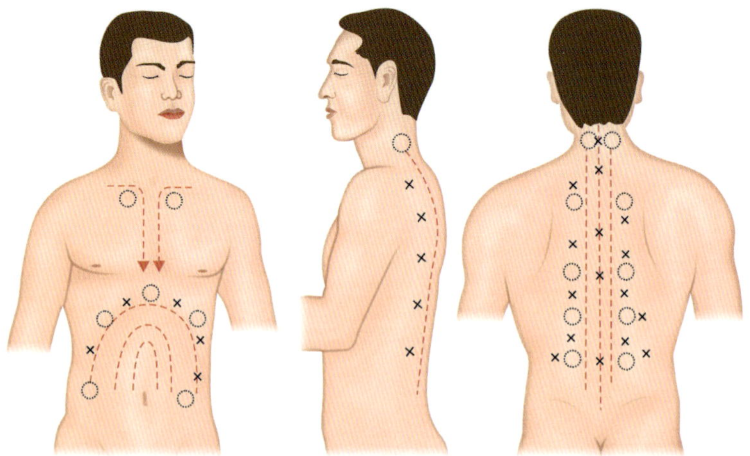

Fig. 62: Insomnia (Localization of injections).

Insufficiency of Cerebral Circulation

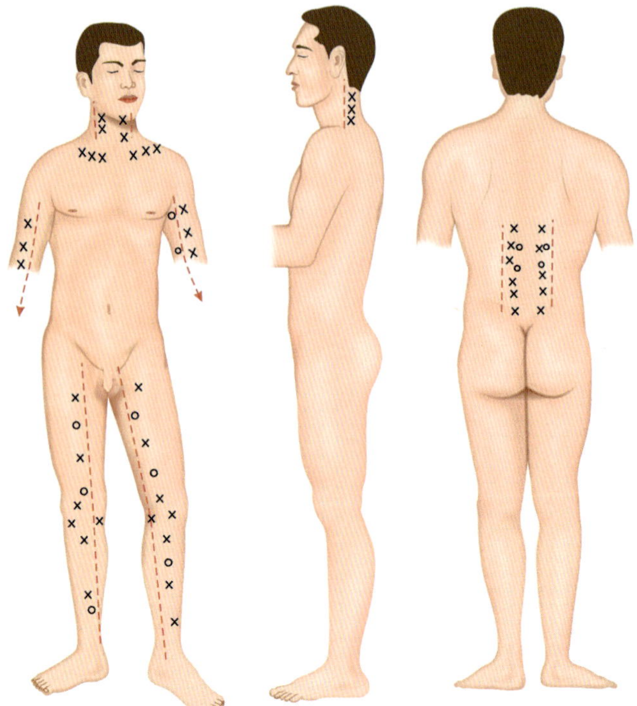

Fig. 63: Insufficiency of cerebral circulation (Localization of injections).

Protocol:

- Xylocaine 0.5%: 1 cc
- Etamsylate: 1 ampule
- Calcitonin 0.50 UI: 1 ampule

Localization (Fig. 63): The injections can be made along the carotid axe, the vascular axes of the superior limbs, and can be completed by a treatment along the inferior limbs; at last it is of a great interest to make some injections along the paravertebral area, especially on the lumbar area which will have the effect of a "chemical sympathectomy", opening the precapillary locks.

The frequency of sessions: D1–D15–D30, and then monthly.

Insufficiency of the Venous Circulation of the Lower Limbs

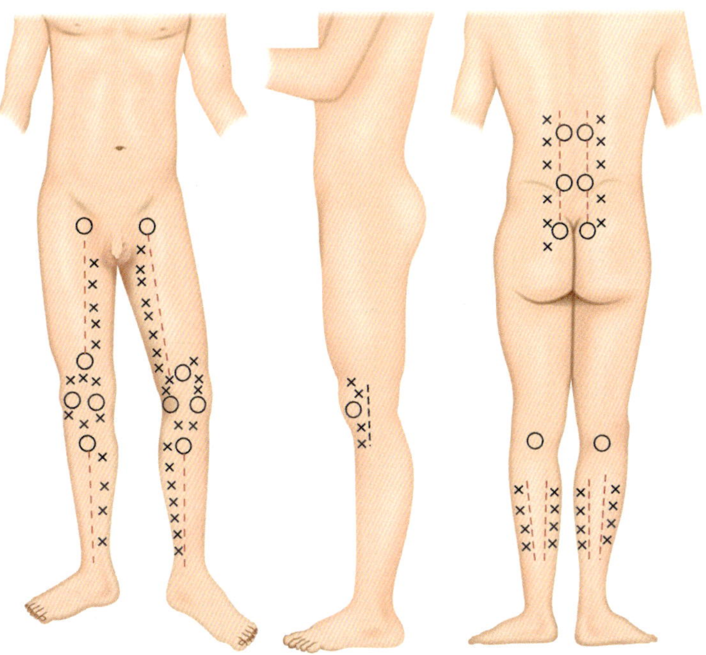

Fig. 64: Insufficiency of the venous circulation of the lower limbs (Localization of injections).

Protocol:

- Xylocaine 0.5%: 1 cc
- Etamsylate: 1 ampule
- Esberiven: 1 ampule.

Localization: Along the vascular axes of the lower limbs, around the knees, and lumbar area (Fig. 64).

Here again it is interesting to treat the lumbar area (effect of chemical sympathectomy).

Frequency: D1–D8–D15, and then monthly.

Knee Arthrosis (Fig. 65)

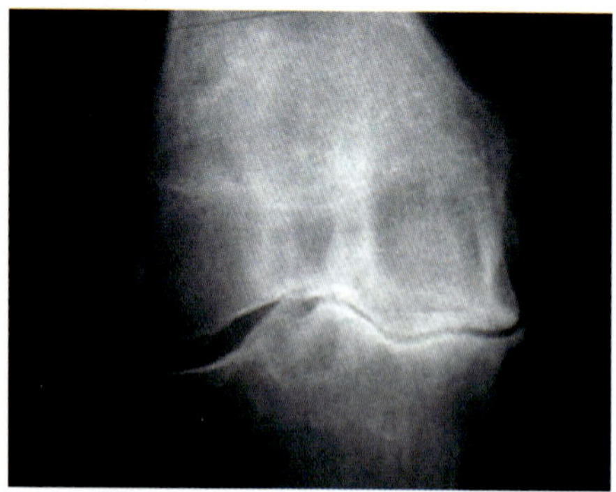

Fig. 65: Knee arthrosis radiography.

Mesotherapy is interesting in this pathology; the best is to begin the treatment the earliest as possible, before a too important evolution of the arthrosis, which would need a surgical approach.

The First Protocol (D1–D7)

It is used in the acute inflammation:

- Xylocaine 0.5% (1 cc)
- Profenid (1 ampule)
- Magnesium (3 cc) for dilution
- Thiocolchicoside (1 ampule)

The Second Protocol (D15–D30)

It is used for chronic period, in order to bring a better vascularization and a regeneration of the area.

- Xylocaine 0.5%: 1 cc
- Etamsylate: 1 ampule
- Calcitonin: 1 ampule (for osteoporosis)
- Magnesium: 3 cc + Thiocolchicoside (1 ampule).

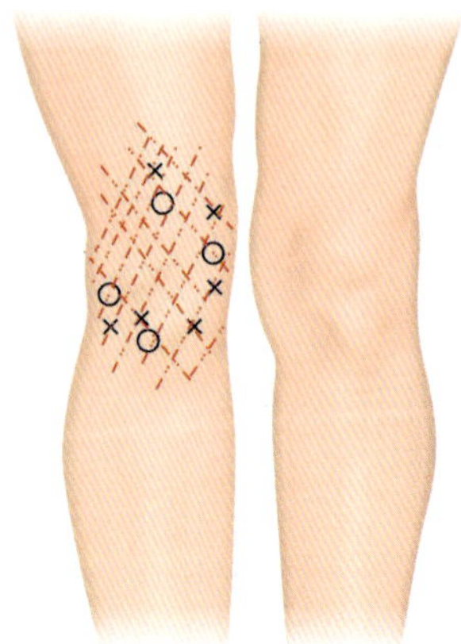

Fig. 66: Knee arthrosis (Localization of injections).

After the two protocols, you can make one session by month with the second protocol. It has a good effect on the general state of the patients, improves mobility, and makes the pain decrease.

Localization (Fig. 66)

Lumbago–Sciatica–Cruralgia

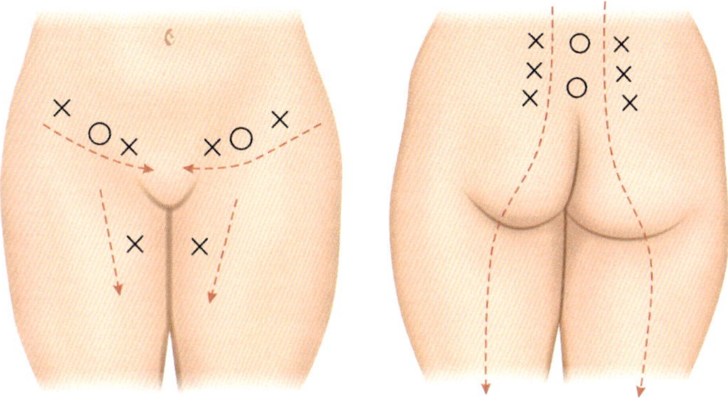

Fig. 67: Lumbago–Cruralgia (Localization of injections).

Protocol

The same protocol used in arthrosis.

- *The first protocol (D1–D7):*
  It is used in the acute inflammation:
  - Xylocaine 0.5% (1 cc)
  - Profenid (1 ampule)
  - Magnesium (3 cc) for dilution
  - Thiocolchicoside (1 ampule)
- *The second protocol (D15–D30):*
  It is used for chronic period, in order to bring a better vascularization and a regeneration of the area.
  - Xylocaine 0.5%: 1 cc
  - Etamsylate: 1 ampule
  - Calcitonin: 1 ampule (for osteoporosis)
  - Magnesium: 3 cc + Thiocholchicosid (1 ampule)

(lumbago-sciatica-cruralgia suite)

Localization (Fig. 67): Make the injections along the vertebral and paravertebral areas, and make continuous injections on the most algic points.

Mastodynia

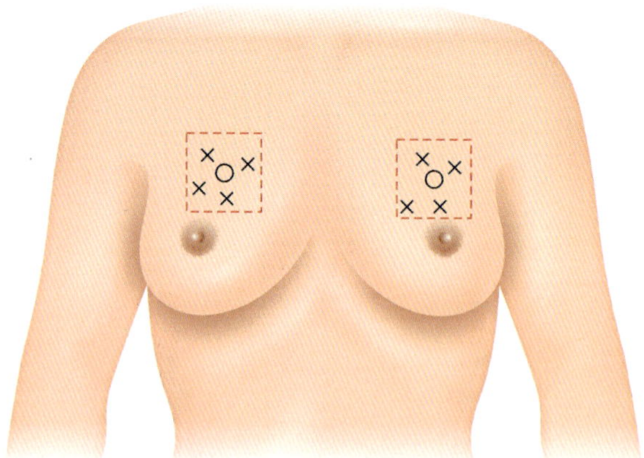

Fig. 68: Mastodynia (Localization of injections).

Mastodynia has different origins, most often linked with mastosis. Mesotherapy can be useful especially with a protocol including vascular treatment.

Protocol (Forbidden if pregnancy, breastfeeding, local infection!!!)

- Xylocaine 5%: 1 cc
- Etamsylate: 1 ampule
- Esberiven: 1 ampule

(If you cannot obtain esberiven, you can replace it with hamamelis and melilot prepared by a homeopathic chemist).

A complementary treatment can be used in the intervals of mesotherapy sessions, for example, local applications of progesterone, after a serious local examination, a proper medical advice, and taking account of the contra-indications.

Localization (Fig. 68)

Frequency: Every 3 months.

Migraine

This is a special part of the treatment of "cephalalgia"; migraine has a specific mesotherapic treatment since we use two particular medications:

- A beta blocker: Avlocardyl
- A vascular medication: Etamsylate or esberiven

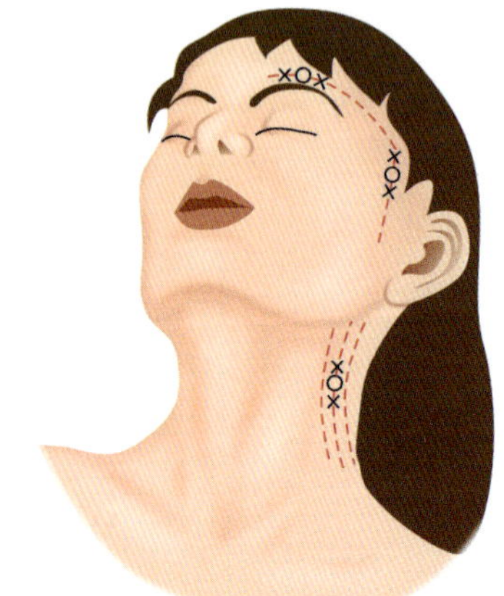

Fig. 69: Migraine (Localization of injections).

It is possible to combine other treatments:
- The protocol of NVD
- A protocol of cervical arthrosis if associated.

Protocol

- Xylocaine 0.5%: 1 cc
- Avlocardyl: 1 ampule
- Etamsylate or esberiven: 1 ampule

Localization (Fig. 69)
Caution: The injections must be subcutaneous, so it is necessary to make a skin fold between the thumb and the index finger, in order to avoid intravascular injection!!!

Neurovegetative Dystonia

This is another very important chapter in mesotherapy treatments; it show the essential place taken by "magnesium" in the treatment of "anxiety" and minor "depressive states". I devoted a great part of my medical activity studying the efficiency of magnesium in those pathologies.

Besides, in our modern world, many patients complain about what they usually call "stress"; this is a very large proportion of our motive of consultations; it is so gratifying to see how the patients feel better with the NVD mesotherapy treatment.

Another benefit is that this kind of treatment helps the patient to reduce the consumption of drugs like anxiolytics, antidepressants, and sleeping drugs.

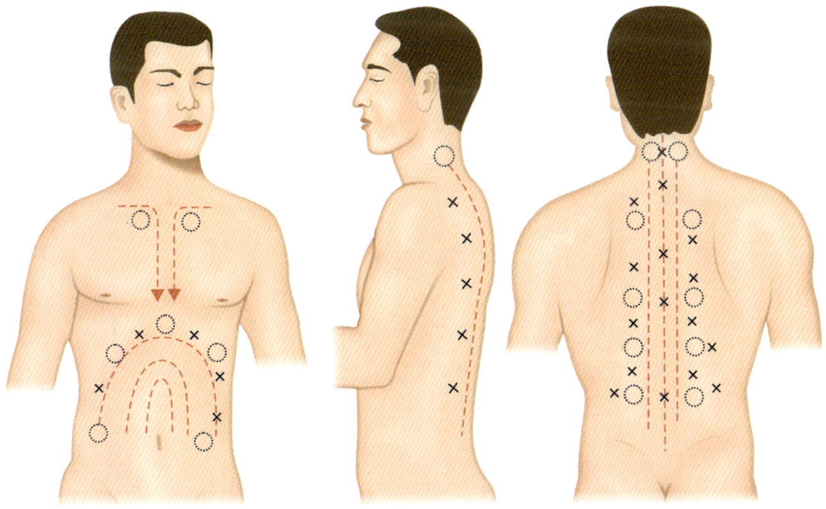

Fig. 70: Neurovegetative dystonia (NDA) (Localization of injections).

Protocol:
- Xylocaine 0.5%: 1 cc
- Thiocolchicoside: 1 ampule
- Mag 2: 3 cc

(Neurovegetative dystonia: suite)

Localization (Fig. 70):
- Subclavicular and sternal areas
- Abdominal area
- Vertebral column area

Frequency: Every month till improvement. It is possible to combine another protocol of stimulation with magnesium and vitamin cocktail, on the same areas.

Neuralgia (Fig. 71)

This part of our work will present three particular indications of mesotherapy:
- *The Arnold's occipital neuralgia*
- *The facial and trigeminal nerve neuralgia*
- *The intercostal neuralgia.*

It is an important chapter of what we could name the *"Pain Management";* a special chapter about this subject will be developed further.

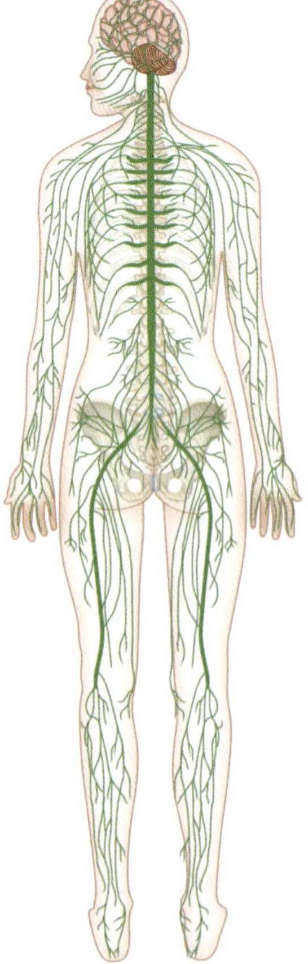

Fig. 71: Neuralgic system.

Arnold's Occipital Neuralgia (Fig. 72)

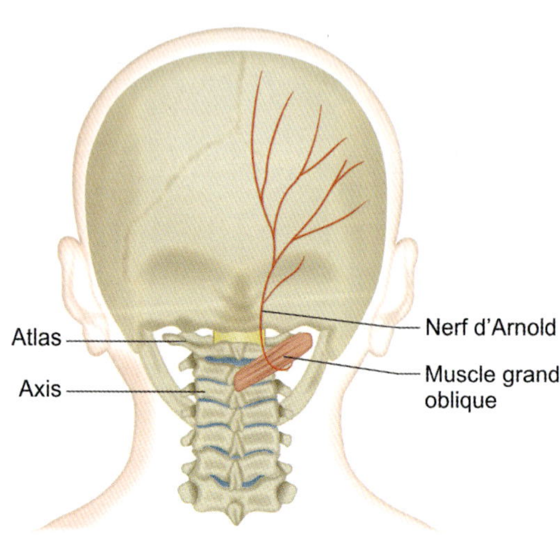

Fig. 72: Arnold's nerve (Nerf d'Arnold).

Occipital neuralgia, also known as *C2 neuralgia,* or (rarely) *Arnold's neuralgia,* is a medical condition characterized by *chronic pain* in the upper neck, back of the head, and behind the eyes. These areas correspond to the locations of the *lesser and greater occipital nerves.* The greater occipital nerve also has an artery that supplies blood that is wrapped around it—the occipital artery, that can contribute to the neuralgia. This condition is also sometimes characterized by diminished sensation in the affected area as well.

Protocol (valid for all types of neuralgia):

- First protocol:
  - Xylocaine 0.5%: 1 cc
  - Etamsylate: 1 ampule
  - B_{12} vitamin (if no contraindication)
- Second protocol:
  - Xylocaine 0.5%: 1 cc
  - Thiocolchicoside: 1 ampule
  - Mag 2: 3 cc

Arnold's neuralgia (suite)

Localization (Fig. 73):

- The injections can be made on the cervico-dorsal areas and reach the shoulder area.
- It also can be useful to treat the muscles of the back: trapezius muscle.
- Large dorsal muscle.

Frequency: D1–D8–D21

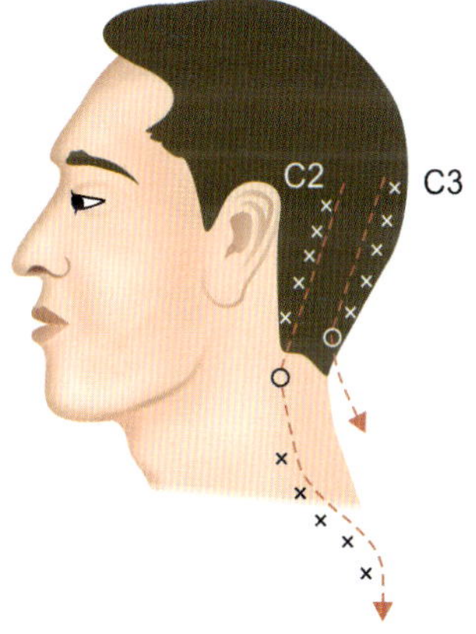

Fig. 73: Arnold's neuralgia (Localization of injections).

FACIAL AND TRIGEMINAL NERVE NEURALGIA

- The anatomy of the trigeminal nerve (Fig. 74)
- The innervation areas (Fig. 75)

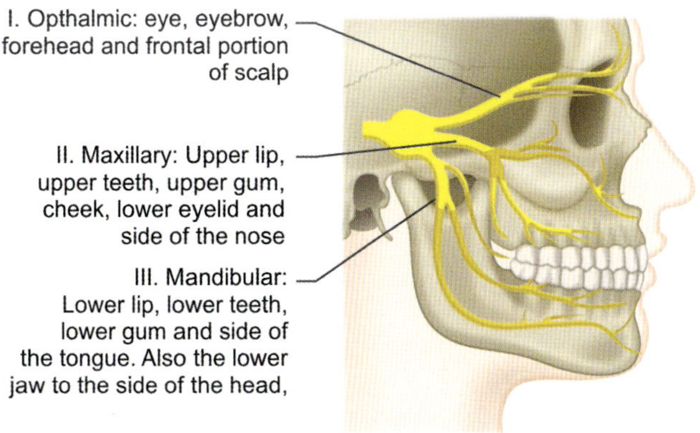

Fig. 74: Trigeminal nerves and its three braches.

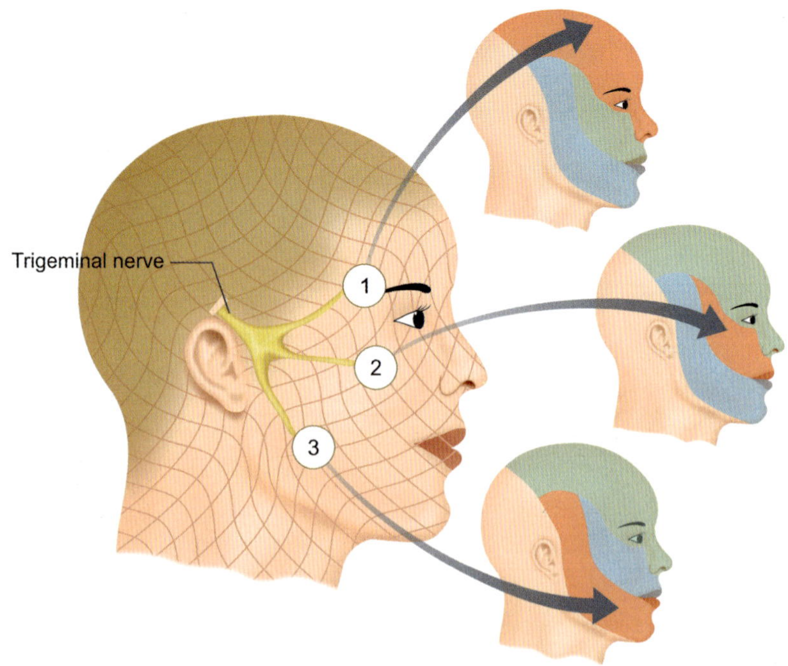

Fig. 75: Trigeminal nerves—innervation areas.

- Trigeminal neuralgia definition: An estimated 1 in 15,000 people have trigeminal neuralgia, also known as *tic douloureux*. It is usually experienced as a severe, stabbing pain to one side of the face, in the eyes, lips, nose, scalp, forehead, jaw or cheek. The pain lasts from a few seconds to a minute or two. Episodes can continue for days, weeks or months, and then disappear for months or years. While the condition is not life-threatening, it is described as among the most painful conditions known, and attacks or fear of attack can be extremely debilitating.

Trigeminal neuralgia occurs most often in people over 50, and more often in women. It may be associated with other disorders, such as multiple sclerosis. The head or face pain is presumed to be caused by a blood vessel pressing the trigeminal nerve as it exits the brainstem. Due to an inherited pattern of blood vessel formation, the condition may run in families.

Trigeminal neuralgia can take time to diagnose because there are many causes of facial pain. In some patients, trigeminal neuralgia is associated with a trigger zone, which can provide one clue for diagnosis. Rather than try to alleviate discomfort by rubbing or applying hot or cold compresses, patients who have a trigger zone tend to avoid activities that are likely to involve that area, such as shaving, biting, chewing, or face washing.

Protocol

- First protocol:
  - Xylocaine 0.5%: 1 cc
  - Etamsylate: 1 ampule
  - B_{12} vitamin (if no contraindication)
- Second protocol:
  - Xylocaine 0.5%: 1 cc
  - Thiocolchicoside: 1 ampule
  - Mag 2: 3 cc

Facial and Trigeminal Neuralgia (suite)

Localization (Fig. 76)

Frequency: D1–D8–D21

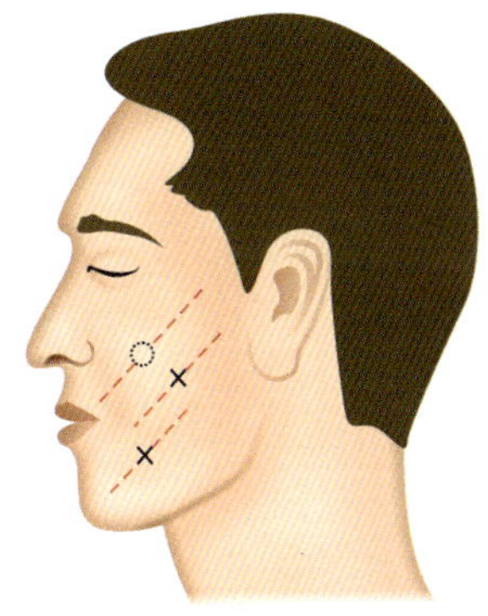

Fig. 76: Trigeminal neuralgia (Localization of injections).

Intercostal Neuralgia

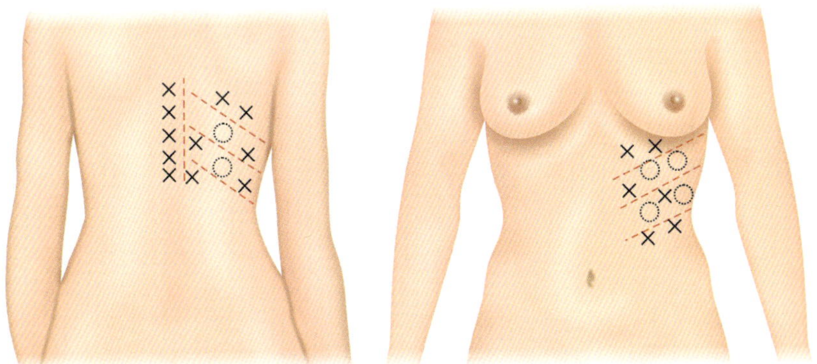

Fig. 77: Intercostal neuralgia (Localization of injections).

Protocol

- First protocol:
  - Xylocaine 0.5%: 1 cc
  - Etamsylate: 1 ampule
  - B_{12} vitamin (if no contraindication)
- Second protocol:
  - Xylocaine 0.5%: 1 cc
  - Thiocolchicoside: 1 ampule
  - Mag 2: 3 cc

Localization (Fig. 77)

Frequency: D1–D8–D21

Osteoporosis (Fig. 78)

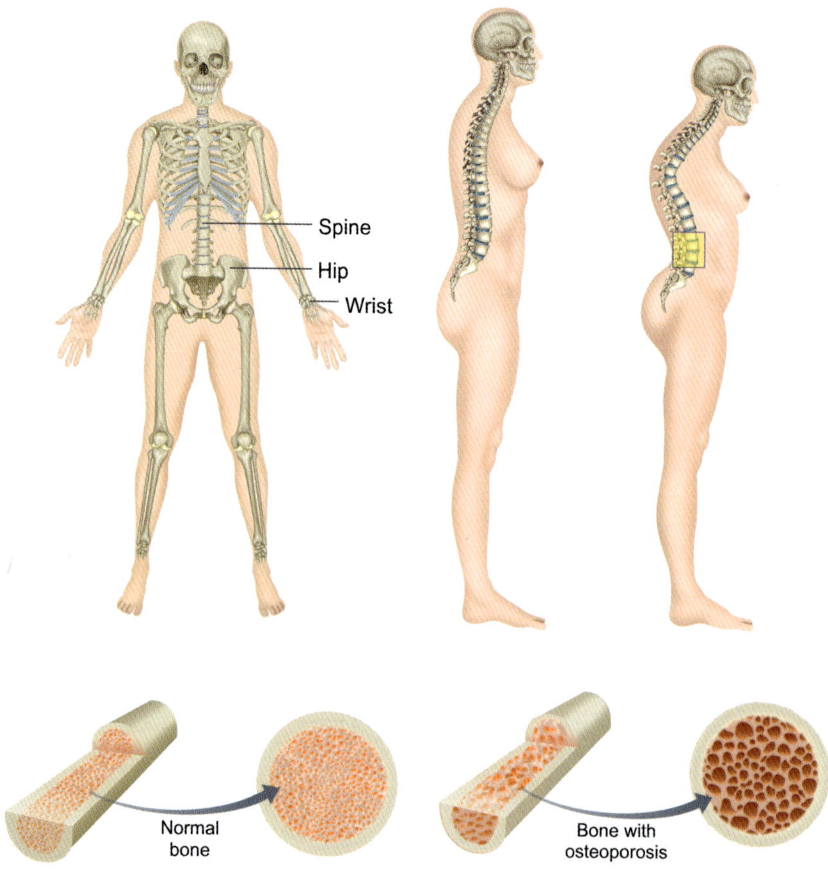

Fig. 78: Osteoporosis.

Definition

Osteoporosis causes bones to become weak and brittle—so brittle that a fall or even mild stresses like bending over or coughing can cause a fracture. Osteoporosis-related fractures most commonly occur in the hip, wrist or spine.

Bone is living tissue that is constantly being broken down and replaced. Osteoporosis occurs when the creation of new bone does not keep up with the removal of old bone.

Osteoporosis affects men and women of all races. But white and Asian women, especially older women who are past menopause, are at highest risk. Medications, healthy diet, and weight-bearing exercise can help prevent bone loss or strengthen already weak bones.

Osteoporosis (suite)

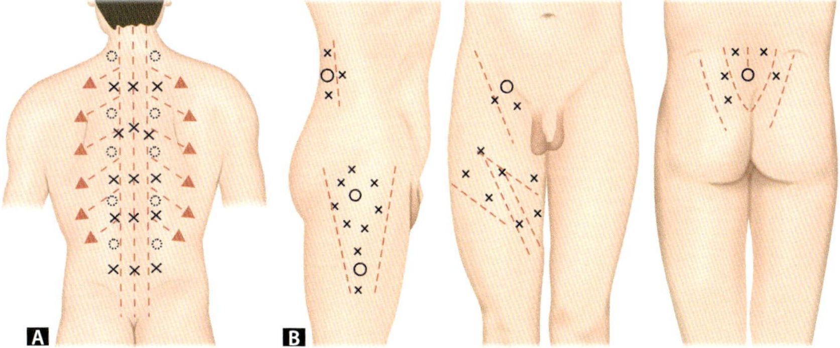

Figs. 79A and B: (A) Vertebral area; (B) Hips and femoral areas.

Symptoms

There typically are no symptoms in the early stages of bone loss. But once bones have been weakened by osteoporosis, you may have signs and symptoms that include:

- Back pain, caused by a fractured or collapsed vertebra
- Loss of height over time
- A stooped posture
- A bone fracture that occurs much more easily than expected.

Protocol:

- Xylocaine 0.5%: 1 cc
- Etamsylate: 1 ampule
- Calcitonin 0.50 UI: 1 ampule

You may alternate with a second protocol:

- Xylocaine 0.5%: 1 cc
- Thiocolchicoside: 1 ampule
- Mag 2: 3 cc

Localization (Figs. 79A and B)

Frequency: D1–D8–D15, and then monthly till improvement.

Periarthritis (Impingement Syndrome)

The Scapulohumeral Periarthritis (Fig. 80)

This pathology has different aspects:

- The simple periarthritis on the scapular area

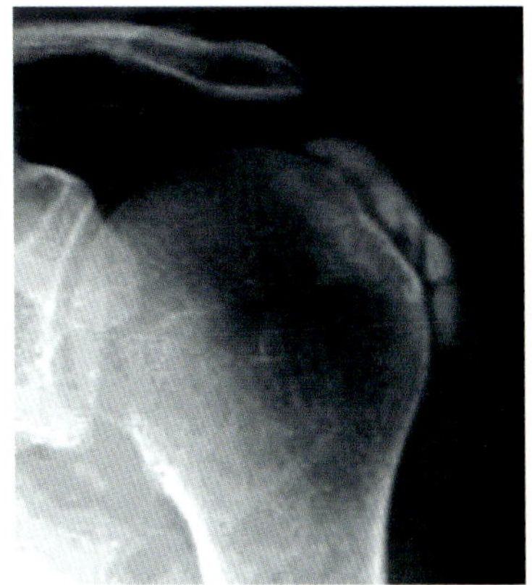

Fig. 80: Periarthritis of the scapula (Radiography)

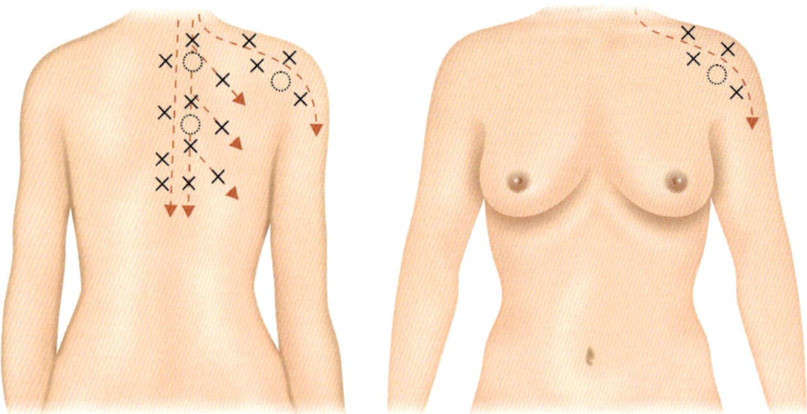

Fig. 81: Periarthritis of the scapula (Localization of injections).

- The periarthritis with *calcification* in the articulation which is more difficult to treat.

In case of simple periarthritis:

The protocol:

- Xylocaine 0.5%: 1 cc
- Diclofenac: 1 ampule
- Mag 2: 3 cc

If a calcification exists in the articulation:

- First step: Local anesthesy of the shoulder area with xylocaine 0.5%: 1 cc. Wait for 5 or 10 minutes.
- Second step: Xylocaine 0.5%: 1 cc; Etamsylate: 1 ampule on the same area.
- Third step: Injection of xylocaine 0.5% 1 cc and tetracemate disodium 1.5 CC (calcium chelator).
  (Cautions*: The injection of tetracemate is very painful, so this is why a local anesthetic protocol is necessary)*

Localization (Fig. 81)

The results are very interesting with a disparition of the calcification in most of the cases.

Presbycusis

Definition

Lessening of hearing acuteness resulting from degenerative changes in the ear that occur especially in old age.

Protocol

- Xylocaine 0.5%: 1 cc

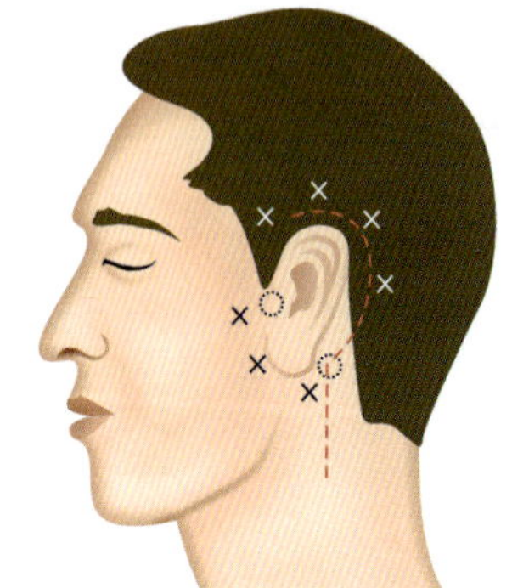

Fig. 82: Presbycusis (Localization of injections).

- Etamsylate: 1 ampule
- Esberiven: 1 ampule

Frequency: Every month

Localization (Fig. 82)

Presbyopia (Farsightedness)

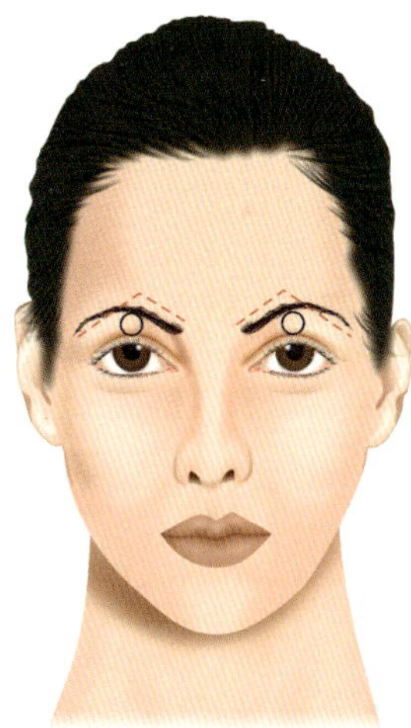

Fig. 83: Presbyopia of the scapula (Localization of injections).

Definition

Presbyopia is the gradual loss of your eyes' ability to focus on nearby objects. It is a natural, often annoying part of aging. Presbyopia usually becomes noticeable in your early to mid-40s and continues to worsen until around age 65.

You may become aware of presbyopia when you start holding books and newspapers at arm's length to be able to read them. A basic eye examination can confirm presbyopia. You can correct the condition with eyeglasses or contact lenses. You might also consider surgery.

Protocol

- Xylocaine 0.5%: 1 cc
- Etamsylate: 1 ampule
- Calcitonin 50 UI: 1 ampule

Frequency: Every 3 months.

Presbyopia (suite)

Localization (Fig. 83)

Caution: The injections must be done very carefully, one point by point on every eyebrow and very fast superficial intradermic injections above the eyebrows.

When injecting, hold the eyebrow between the thumb and the index, the injection is easier to perform with the mesogun.

Raynaud's Disease (Fig. 84)

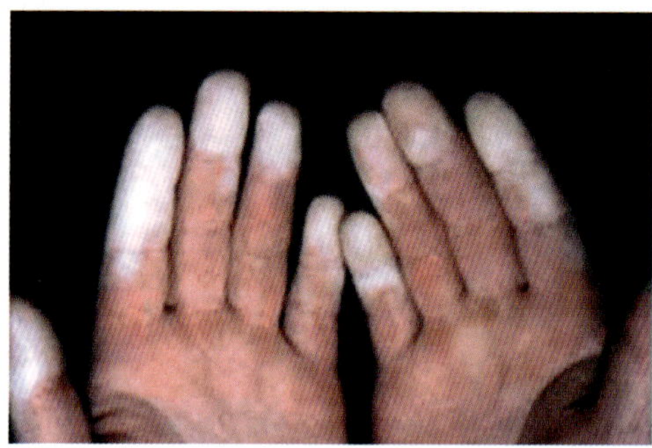

Fig. 84: Raynaud's disease.

Raynaud's disease causes some areas of your body, such as your fingers and toes, to feel numb and cold in response to cold temperatures or stress. In Raynaud's disease, smaller arteries that supply blood to your skin narrow, limiting blood circulation to affected areas (vasospasm).

Women are more likely than men to have Raynaud's disease, also known as Raynaud or Raynaud's phenomenon or syndrome. It appears to be more common in people who live in colder climates.

Protocol:

- Xylocaine 0.5%: 1 cc
- Etamsylate: 1 ampule
- Calcitonin 0.50 UI: 1 ampule

Rhythm of sessions: D1-D7-D15-D30 and once a month, in the cold period of weather.

Raynaud's disease (suite)

Localization: It can be interesting to complete with injections on the lumbar area (Fig. 85).

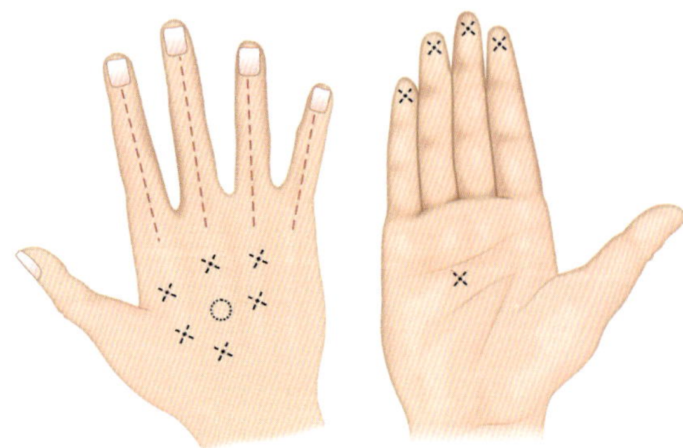

Fig. 85: Raynaud's disease (Localization of injections).

Rhinitis (Allergic Rhinitis)

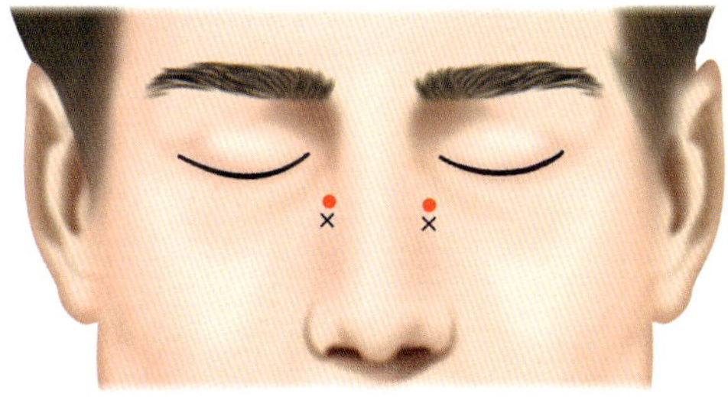

Fig. 86: Rhinitis (Localization of injections).

Protocol:

- Xylocaine 0.5% (1 cc)
- Polaramine: 1 ampule (antiallergic)
- Magnesium (1 cc)

Rhythm of the sessions: D1–D7–D15

Localization (Fig. 86).

Rhizarthrosis (Fig. 87)

In rhizarthrosis, the osteoarthritic lesions are located at the joint between the first metacarpal and the wrist bone (the trapezium). This is osteoarthritis of the trapeziometacarpal joint. This joint allows a movement known as "opposition of the thumb". This joint allows you to put your thumb in opposition to your other fingers. This is the joint that comes into play in "pinching" movements (thumb and index finger, thumb and little finger, etc.).

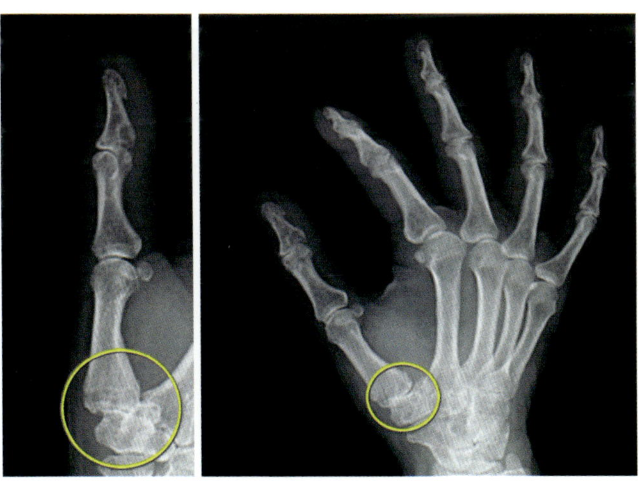

Fig. 87: Rhizarthrosis radiography.

In the long-term, an affected joint determines:

- A "Z-shaped" deformation of the thumb at the joint
- A reduction in volume of the muscles of the palm of the hand (those in the extension of the thumb).

Rhizarthrosis (suite)

Protocol

- The first protocol (D1–D7): It is used in the acute inflammation.
  - Xylocaine 0.5 % (1 cc)
  - Profenid (1 ampule)
  - Magnesium (3 cc) for dilution
- The second protocol (D15–D30): It is used for chronic period, in order to bring a better vascularization.
  - Xylocaine 0.5%: 1 cc
  - Etamsylate: 1 ampule
  - Calcitonin: 1 ampule (for osteoporosis).

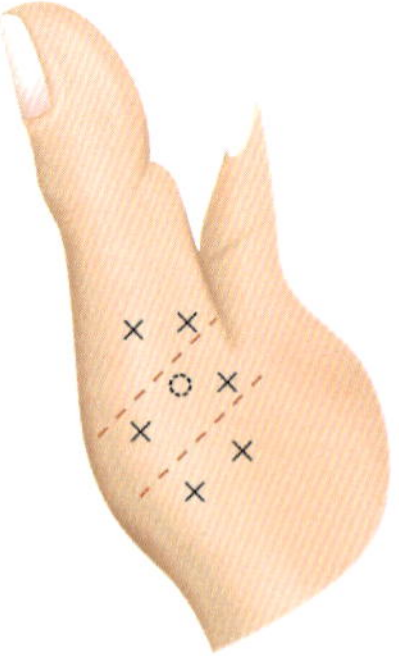

Fig. 88: Rhizarthrosis (Localization of injections).

Frequency: Every month.

Localization (Fig. 88)

Sinusitis (Chronic Sinusitis) (Fig. 89)

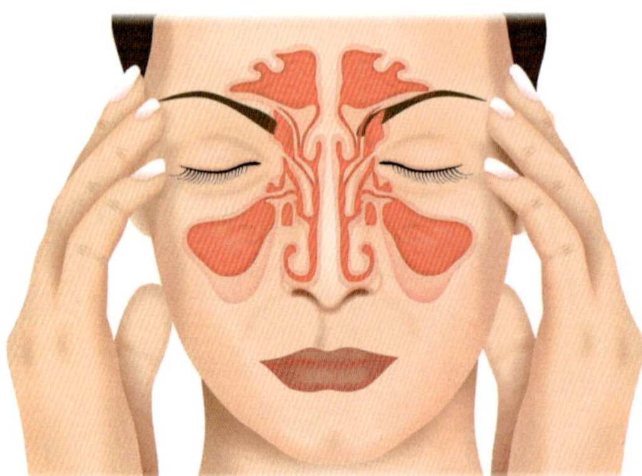

Fig. 89: Sinusitis.

In this chapter we only talk about the chronic sinusitis which can be treated with the protocol of immunostimulation.

Sprain of the Ankle (Fig. 90)

In this indication, we only consider the treatment of the minor sprains, after having made a serious clinic examination (and radiologic examination, if necessary).

No intervention must be done in the very first 24–48 hours the sprain occurs, after local ice applications, elastic contention, and walking aid.

Frequency: D1–D8–D15

Protocol:

- Xylocaine 0.5%: 1 cc
- Etamsylate: 2 cc
- Arnica 4DH: 1–3 cc

Localization (Fig. 91).

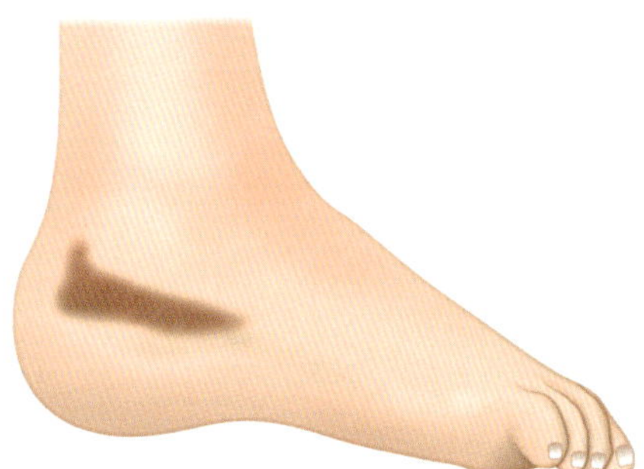

Fig. 90: Sprain of the ankle.

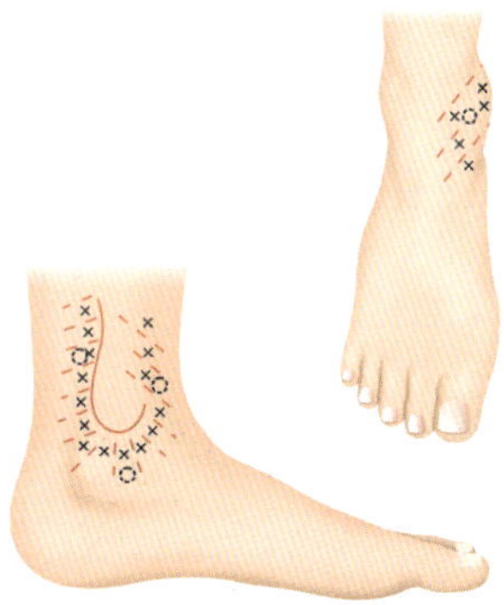

Fig. 91: Sprain (Localization of injections).

Synovial Cyst (Fig. 92)

A synovial cyst is a small, fluid-filled sac or pouch that can develop over a tendon or joint, creating a mass under the skin. Synovial cysts are found most commonly in the wrist, knee, and hip. Cysts also can form in the shoulder, elbow, hand (flexor tendon sheath in the fingers), top of the foot (dorsum), and ankle. A synovial cyst may or may not be painful, depending on their size and location.

Protocol:

- Xylocaine 0.5%: 1 cc
- Etamsylate: 1 cc
- Magnesium: 2 cc

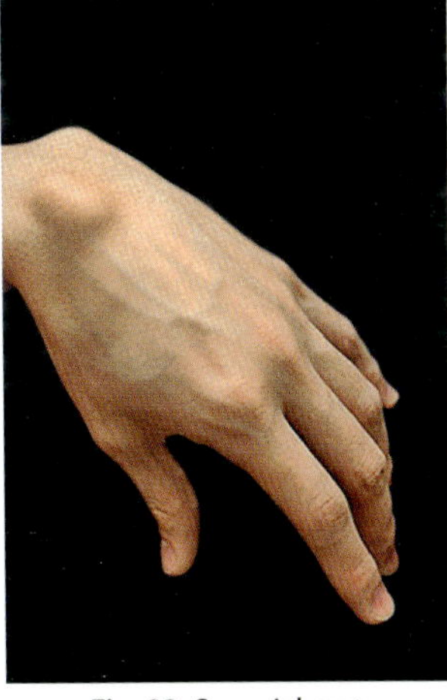

Fig. 92: Synovial cyst.

Localization (Figs. 93 and 94):

- Use continuous injections:
  - One in the center of the cyst
  - Four injections in the cardinal points of the cyst.

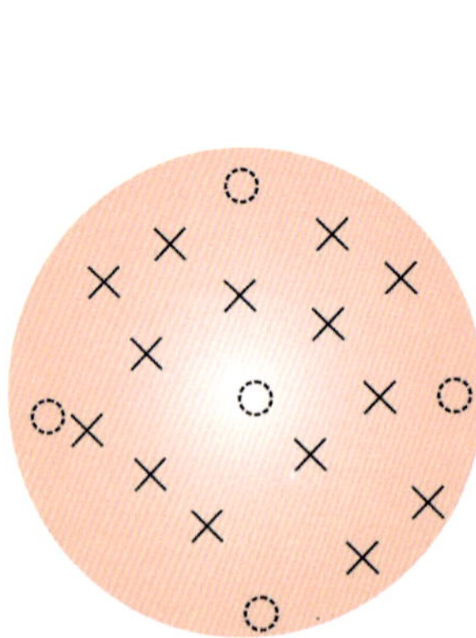

Fig. 93: Synovial cyst: The four injections at the cardinal points.

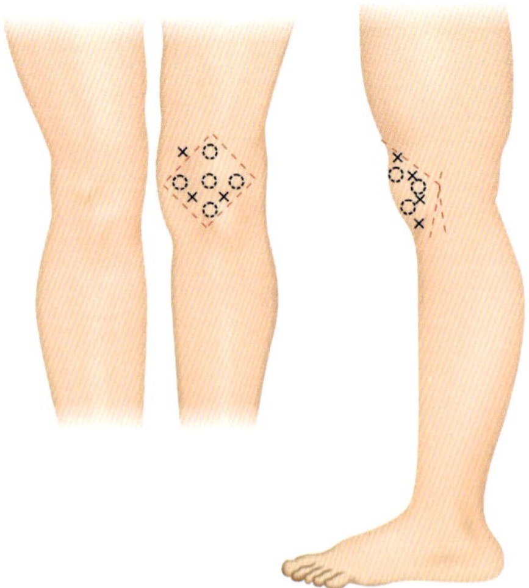

Fig. 94: Synovial cyst of the knee (Localization of injections).

Synovial cyst (suite)

- You can complete with superficial injections all around the cyst.
- This technique is worthwhile for the different localizations of the cyst.

Frequency of sessions: Monthly

Caution: *One exception is the cyst of the popliteal space in which you must not make deep injections; there is a risk of intervascular injection!*

The same caution has to be observed in radial localization of the cyst.

Talalgia (Calcaneal Spur) (Fig. 95)

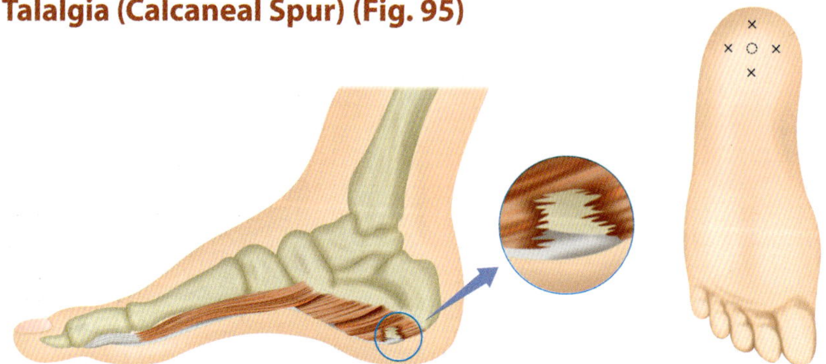

Fig. 95: Talalgia.

Fig. 96: Talalgia (Localization of injections).

Protocol:
- Xylocaine 0.5%: 1 cc
- Etamsylate: 1 ampule
- Magnesium: 2 cc

Frequency: D1–D15–D30

Localization: Be cautious, the injection is painful, and it may be useful to prepare the area of injection by local application of anesthetic like a patch of "EMLA" (Fig. 96).

Tendinitis (Achilles Tendinitis) (Fig. 97)

The Achilles tendinitis is important to treat the most precociously as possible. In case of tendinitis, the tendon is fragile and can break; a mesotherapy treatment has many interesting effects on the tendon:
- Increasing the microcirculation
- Improving the healing of the tendon
- Preventing the Achilles tendon rupture.

The diagnosis of the rupture can be made with the "Thompson test" (Fig. 98).

(Achilles tendinitis: suite)

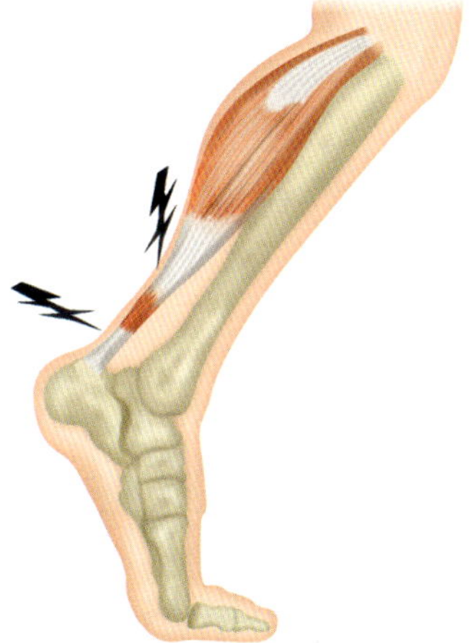

Fig. 97: Tendinitis.

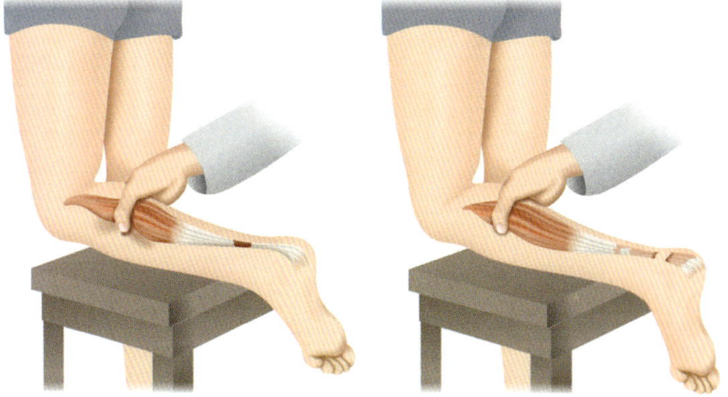

Squeezing the calf muscles causes them to contract, thus plantar flexion will occur, However, if no plantar flexion occurs, the Achilles tendon is ruptured

Fig. 98: The Thompson test.

Protocol:

- Inflammation protocol:
  - Xylocaine 0.5% (1 cc)
  - Profenid (1 ampule)
  - Magnesium (3 cc) for dilution
  - Thiocolchicoside (1 ampule)
- Chronic period:
  - Xylocaine 0.5%: 1 cc
  - Etamsylate: 1 ampule
  - Calcitonin: 1 ampule.

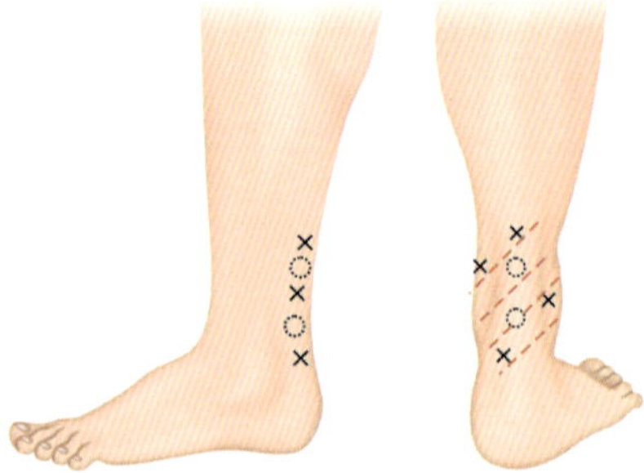

Fig. 99: Tendinitis (Localization of injections).

Frequency:

- D1: Protocol of inflammation
- D7–D15–D30: Protocol of chronic period.

Localization (Fig. 99)

Zona (Herpes Zoster) (Fig. 100)

This is a good indication of mesotherapy; here again it is important to treat at the very beginning of the pathology; and it helps preventing the zosterian pain which is so unbearable, especially for elderly patients.

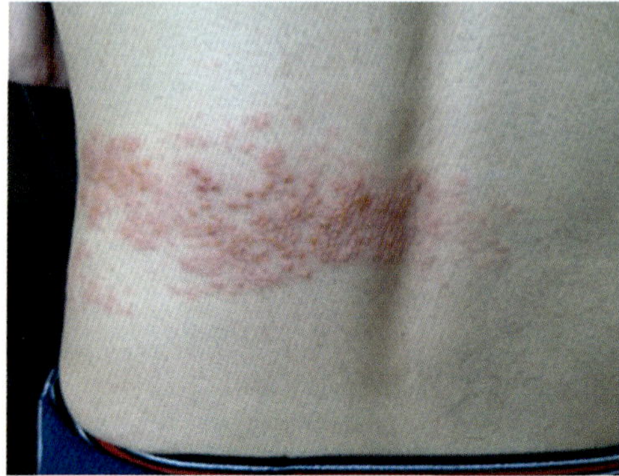

Fig. 100: Zona.

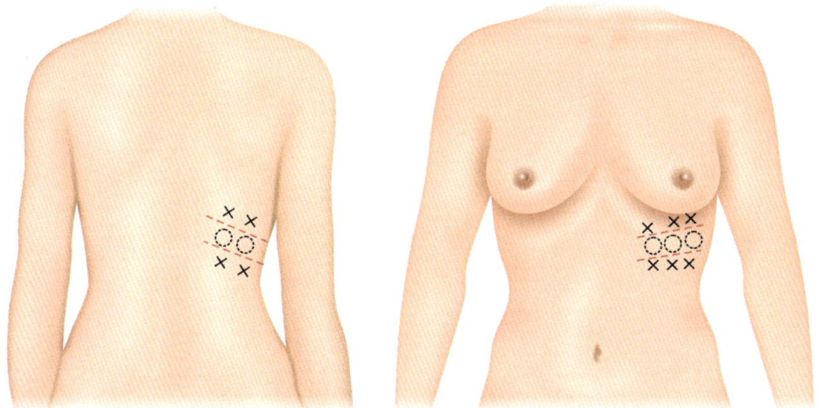

Fig. 101: Zona (Localization of injections).

Of course, the classic antiviral allopathic therapy has to be associated with mesotherapy.

Protocol:

- Xylocaine 0.5%: 1 cc
- Thiocolchicoside: 1 ampule
- Vitamin B_{12}: 2 cc.

It can be interesting to alternate with the immunostimulation protocol.

Frequency: D1–D8–D15 and when needed.

Localization (Fig. 101):

10

THE PAIN MANAGEMENT

In this chapter, we will see the pathologies in which the pain is always manifested. Some indications have been already mentioned, some others will be developed; mesotherapy brings a very helpful contribution to the pain relief.

Definition of Pain

"Pain is a sensorial experiment, emotional, unpleasant, associated with a real or potential lesion of the tissues, described in terms mentioning that lesion"

—International Association of Pain Study

The three components of the pain:

1. The nociceptive component: Aggression → stimulation of peripheric receptors → painful response.
2. The neurogenic component: The neurogenic pain corresponds to a partial or total alteration of the peripheric or central nervous system → neuropathic pains
3. The psychogenic component.

The Pain Tracks

From aggression to cerebral integration.

Theory of physiological control of pain based on the proposal that pain impulses are mediated in the substantia gelatinosa of the spinal cord and the dorsal horns act as "gates" that control the entry of pain signals into the central pain pathways (Figs. 102 and 103).

Gate Control and Mesotherapy

- The prick of the needle induces mechanisms of "Gate Control".
- The nociceptive impulses can be neutralized at the level of the medullar interneuron by stimulating the beta fibers (tact receptors).
- Mesotherapy could stimulate the beta fibers of big caliber which activate the gate control.
- This is a beneficial and short reaction, involving the medullar circuit, and probably intervening in the mesotherapy action.

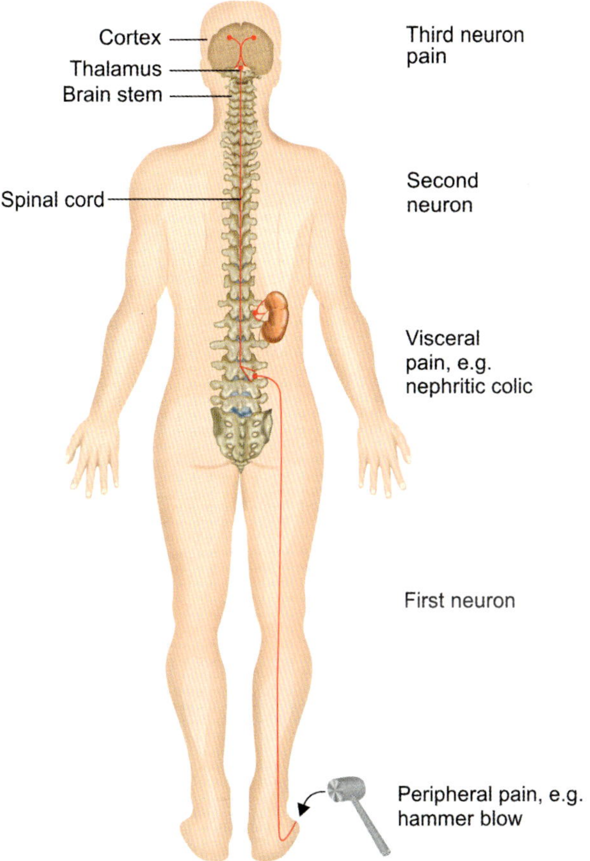

Fig. 102: The gate control system.

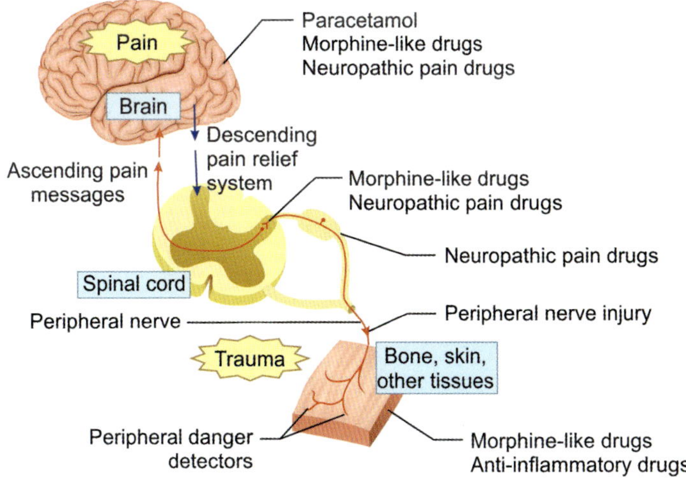

Fig. 103: Brain pain management system.

What Kind of Pain for a Mesotherapy Treatment?

- Visceral pains: Gynecologic, intestinal, urologic
- Cancerology: Metastatic pains
- Vascular pains: Arteritis, venous insufficiency
- Dermatologic pains: Zona
- Neurologic pains: Neuropathic pains, headache, hemicrania
- Rheumatologic pains: Acute and chronical pains
- Sport injuries.

What Drugs Do We Use in Mesotherapy for Pain Treatments?

Visceral Pains

- Myorelaxant: Magnesium (Mag 2, Spasmag)
- Antispasmodic: Phloroglucinol (Spasfon)
- Thiocolchicoside (Miorel and coltramyl).

Cancerology (Fig. 104)

Metastatic pains

- Antalgic drugs:
  - Acetic salicylic acid: Aspirin
  - Nefopam chlorhydrate: Acupan

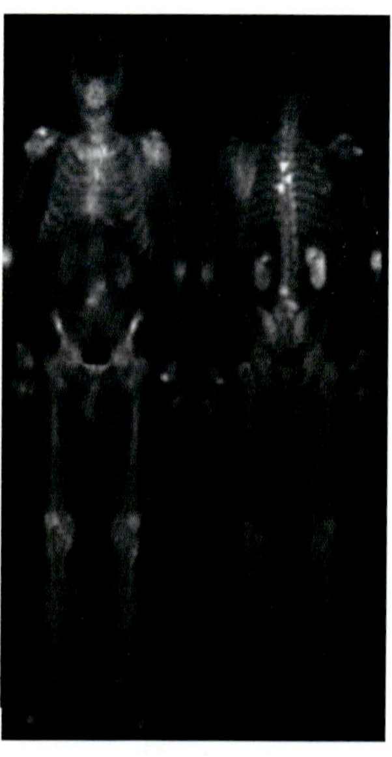

Fig. 104: Bone metastases (Radiography).

Vascular Pains

- Arteritis: The antalgic effect is due to two kinds of drugs: Vasodilatators: Etamsylate, dicynone, and pentoxifylline (Torental)
- Venous insufficiency: Etamsylate and arnica.

Dermatologic Pain: Zona (Fig. 105)

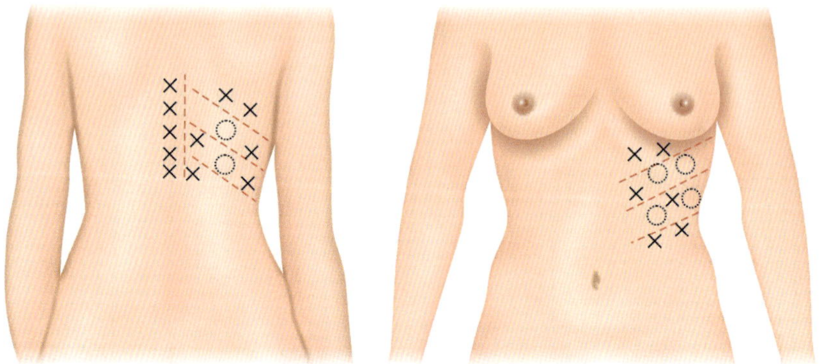

Fig. 105: Zona (Localization of injections).

The antalgic protocol:

- Xylocaine 0.5%: 1 cc
- Thiocolchicoside: 1 ampule
- B_{12} vitamin: 1 ampule

Neurologic Pains

Neuropathic pains:

We can use:

- B_{12} vitamin
- Thiocolchicoside
- Magnesium
- Acupan (Nefopam chlorhydrate).

Rheumatologic Pains

- *The first protocol (D1–D7):*

  It is used in the acute inflammation:
  - Xylocaine 0.5% (1 cc)
  - Profenid (1 ampule)
  - Magnesium (3 cc) for dilution
  - Thiocolchicoside (1 ampule).
- *The second protocol (D15–D30):*

It is used for chronic period, in order to bring a better vascularization, and a regeneration of the vertebral area.

- Xylocaine 0.5%: 1 cc
- Etamsylate: 1 ampule
- Calcitonin: 1 ampule (for osteoporosis)
- Magnesium 3 cc + Thiocolchicoside (1 ampule).

After the two protocols, you can make one session by month with the second protocol. It has a good effect on the general state of the patients, improves mobility, and makes the pain decrease.

The localizations depend on the different pathologies.

It is a good thing to associate different therapeutics:

- Anti-arthrosis medications
- Vitamins
- Oligotherapy
- Homeopathy—acupuncture
- Physiotherapy.

Sports Injuries (Fig. 106)

In sport traumatology:

- Anti-inflammation drugs: Ketoprofen (tendinitis, acute lumbago)
- Myorelaxing drugs: Thiocolchicoside, magnesium (muscle contraction)
- Calcitonin: Especially in algodystrophy
- Etamsylate (sprains).

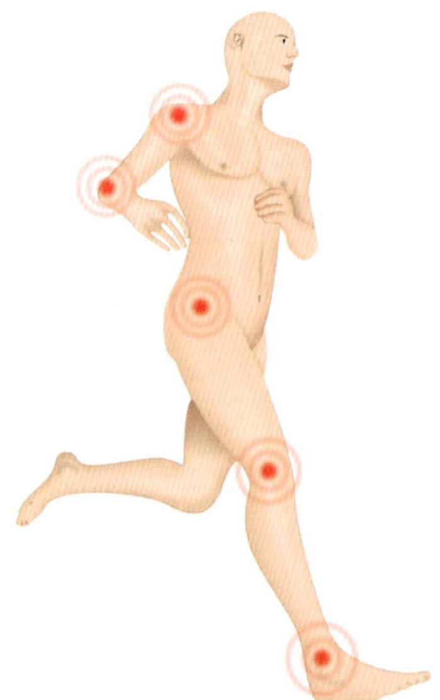

Fig. 106: Sports injuries.

11

MESOTHERAPY APPLICATIONS IN AESTHETIC

This chapter is about some interesting applications in aesthetic; it is important to be aware of the different techniques and medications applied in this particular field of applications, and I suggest to my young colleagues to have a specific training with some specialist in this discipline.

Indeed, there are particular risks in aesthetic; the facial treatments are delicate, and some drugs must be used with special care and precision.

There is also a specific issue related to the important requests of some patients who ask for an unreasonable number of sessions, especially in facial treatments, cellulite, or fat problems.

This is the responsibility of the practitioner to set the rules adapted for each case.

These are the indications we will develop in this chapter:

- Hair loss management
- Cellulite
- Vascular pathology
- Dermatologic pathologies
- Mesolift
- Scars and stretch marks.

In aesthetic treatment, we will have the benefits of the mesotherapy effects, particularly on the skin:

- Local action of medicine
- Diffusion of medications via superficial and deep vasculature
- Stimulation of the superficial and deep dermal plexus.

Let us recall the mesotherapy techniques of injection, and their interest in aesthetic mesotherapy:

- Intraepidermal
- Papular
- Nappage
- Point by point.

Intraepidermal (1 mm):

- Applied on the epidermis
- Painless, no bleeding
- Stimulation of the skin
- Rapid onset of action
- Large surfaces covered

This technique can be applied in the “mesolift” treatment.

Papular (4 mm):

- Injection to the epidermodermal junction
- Lifting of epidermis from basal layer
- Painful.

This technique can be applied for "scalp treatments".

Nappage (2–4 mm) (Fig. 107):

- Continuous
- 2–4 manual injections per second
- Depth of 2–4 mm
- Injection angle 30–60 degrees
- Stimulation of skin
- Rapid onset of action.

  This technique can be applied on "scalp and large cellulite treatments".

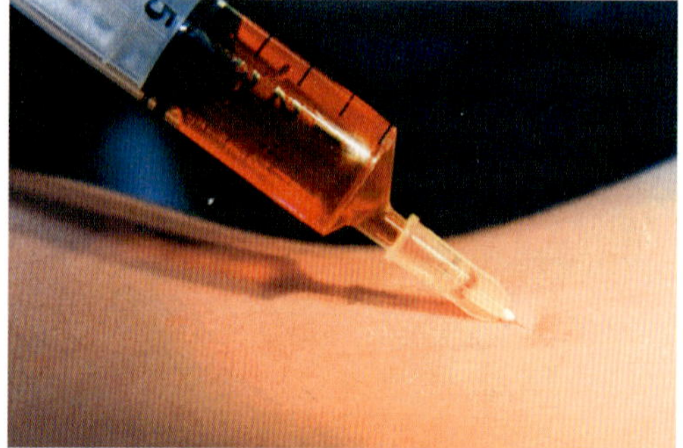

Fig. 107: Nappage.

Point by point (4 mm) (Fig. 108):

- Precise single injections into deep dermis/subcutaneous
- Little pain when product is been delivered
- Commonly used.

This technique can be applied in "fat reduction and cellulite treatments".

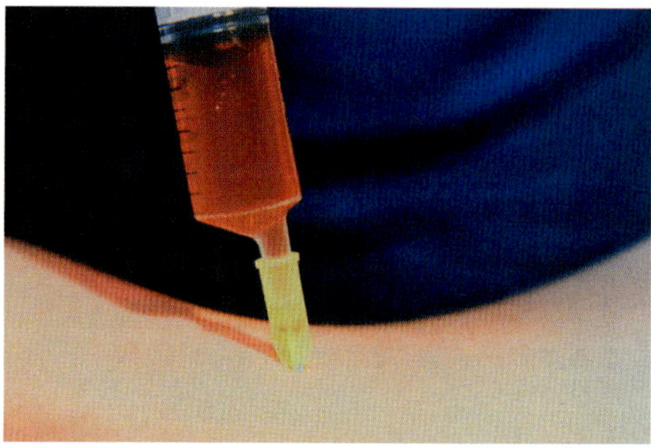

Fig. 108: Point by point.

Aesthetic Mesotherapy: What is Required?

These are the things every therapist should have:

- Sterilizing solution
- Gauze-cotton wool
- Gloves
- 5 cc and 10 cc syringes
- 27G/30G needles
- Injection products
- Mesogun.

(*You can report to the chapter: Mesotherapy equipment-material)*

Contraindications in Aesthetic Mesotherapy

In aesthetic mesotherapy, the contraindications are those of classic mesotherapy.

On the other hand, some medications have their specific side effects and must be perfectly known by the practitioner.

Contraindications:

- Absolute contraindications:
  - Pregnancy
  - Known intolerance or allergy
  - Predisposition to hypertrophic scars or pigmentation disorders
  - Highly active autoimmune process
  - Severe cardiovascular or metabolic disorder
  - Acute viral or bacterial infection
  - Acute inflammatory skin condition
  - Epilepsy.
- Relative contraindications:
  - Age below 16 years
  - Breastfeeding mothers
  - Injection phobia
  - Herpes simplex virus (HSV1), preventive treatment with an antiviral agent (acyclovir or valaciclovir) is advisable
  - Coagulation anomalies or anticoagulation (for deep injection techniques)
  - Existed or suspected destruction of anatomical structure
  - Dysmorphophobia or dysmorphic syndrome *(Distorted perception of one's body).*

Before the Treatment: The Consultation

Before every treatment, it is important to observe the rules of classic medical consultation:

- History, inspection, palpation, and marking the skin
- Observation criteria:
  - Face, frontal, overview

- Face, side view, profile
- Body, overall view, front, back, side views

- Key points of the first consultation:
  - Marking
  - Objectivization and documentation
  - Informing the patient of before and after rules.

Before Beginning

Some Warnings about Aesthetic Medications

All the medications presented in this book are those we use in France; in other countries in Europe and Asia, you can find some pre-prepared "cocktails" and many preparations which are not authorized in France.

Remember: *No more than three products in a syringe!*

Another medication we do not use is the "Lipostabil" (phosphatidylcholine and deoxycholate); this drug used for fatness is forbidden in France; there are side effects (reddening, swelling, pain, and nodules formation), and we have some other medications which can be used with no risk.

Besides, we will not talk about the "Botox" treatments; this is a special part of facial treatment and must be taught by specialists well-aware of the specific uses and risks of this drug.

In the next chapters, we shall present:

- The aesthetic applications of mesotherapy
- The medications used for every case
- The rhythm of the sessions for every indication.

12

ALOPECIA AND MESOTHERAPY (HAIR LOSS)

Figure 109 shows the alopecia and mesotherapy (hair loss).

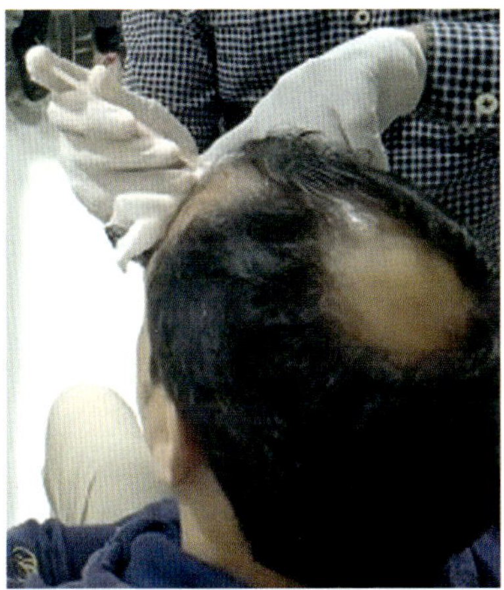

Fig. 109: Scalp mesotherapy.

Normal values:

- Growth: 1 cm/month
- Length of life of one hair: 2–5 years
- Length of one hair: Max 75 cm
- Hair cycles during a life time: Max 25–30
- Maximal constraint of one hair: 100 g
- Scalp: 80,000–150,000 hair
- Density: 180–350 hair/cm^2
- Rate of hair loss: 50–70 hair a day
- Thickness of hair: 0.07 mm.

Classification of Alopecia

- Androgenic alopecia
- Diffuse alopecia
- Alopecia areata
- Scarring alopecia.

Androgenic Alopecia

Definition: Loss of hair occurring in both sex, linked with the stimulation of the hair follicle by androgens. The predilection areas of androgenic alopecia are the frontotemporal area and the vertex.

Etiology (Fig. 110)

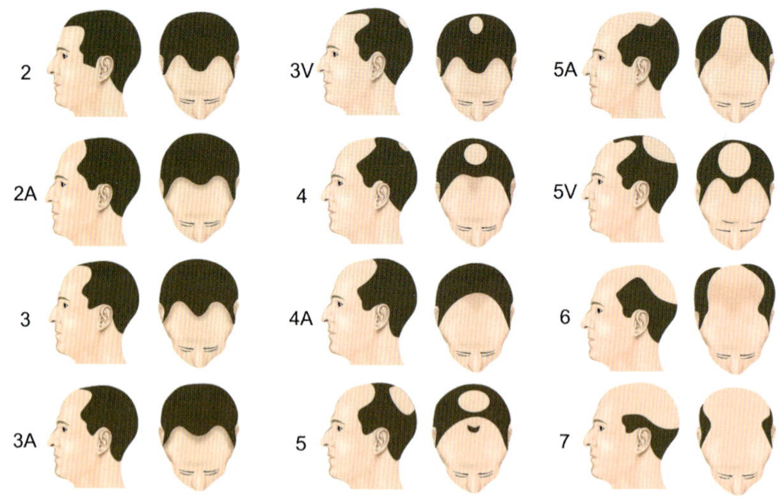

Fig. 110: Various stages of alopecia.

- Aging
- Adrenal hyperplasia
- Syndrome of polycystic ovaries
- Ovarian hyperplasia
- Carcinoid tumors
- Hypophyseal dysfunction
- Drugs: Testosterone, danazol, adrenocorticotropic hormone, anabolic steroids, progesterone.

Diffuse Alopecia (Fig. 111)

Definition: Loss of more than 100 hairs during more than 3 months.

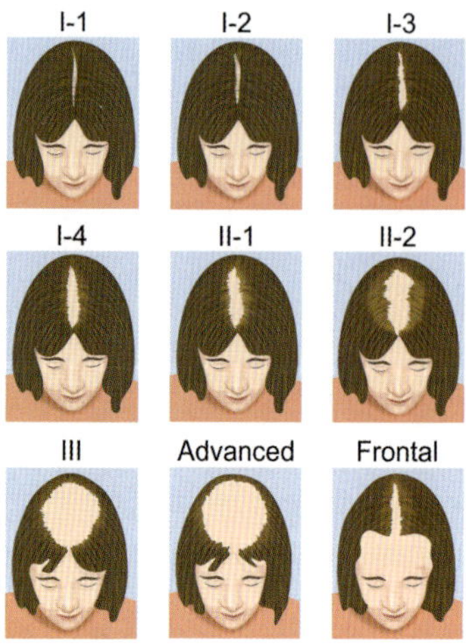

Fig. 111: Women: Various stages of alopecia.

Etiologies:

- Drugs: Cytostatics, anticoagulants, high blood pressure treatments, and antidepressants
- Chronic diseases (influenza, typhus, hepatitis, and tuberculosis)
- Endocrinous pathologies: hypothyroidism, hyperthyroidism, and diabetes
- Effluvium of postpartum
- Nutritional deficiency.

Alopecia Areata

Causes:

- Unknown cause, psychosomatic participation?
- Occurs generally to patients having an autoimmune disease, e.g. thyroidism or pernicious anemia.

Treatment (medical classic treatment):

- Induction of contact sensibilization
- Diphenylcyclopropenone (diphencyprone, DCP)
- Dibutyl squaric acid (SADBE)
- Nonspecific irritating products
- Anthralin 0.5%
- Psoralen and ultraviolet A (PUVA) therapy
- Corticoids
- Cyclosporine A.

Scarring Alopecia (Cicatricial Alopecia)

Definition: Scarring alopecia is a diverse group of rare disorders that destroy the hair follicle, replace it with scar tissue, and cause permanent hair loss.

Etiologies

- Genetic disease (ectodermic dysplasia)
- Infection: Leprosy, syphilis, zona, leishmaniasis
- Basocellular carcinoma
- Traumatic, post-surgery
- Epidermic nevus
- Physical agent: Acid and alkaline, burn, sequela of cryotherapy, and radiodermitis
- Cicatricial pemphigoid
- Lichen planus
- Sarcoidosis.

Mesotherapic Management of Alopecia

Mesotherapy is a therapeutic option between *systemic therapies* (e.g. oral medications) and the *external therapies* (e.g. topic applications).

Active pharmacologic substances are directly injected in the concerned capillary areas.

The advantage: Mesotherapy allows the optimization of the pharmacologic action of the drugs injected in the capillary area, while minimizing the general side effects.

Like every mesotherapy session:

- Medical file: Questioning, medical history, and allergy
- Clinic examination
- Ask biological check-up: Blood numeration, sedimentation rate, ferritin, and thyroid-stimulating hormone.

In doubt about any endocrinous pathology or any else pathology, ask for a specialist advice before beginning mesotherapy!

You have to eliminate every serious disease!

Indications:

- Androgenic male alopecia (Fig. 112):
  - Postpartum effluvium
  - Post-chemotherapy

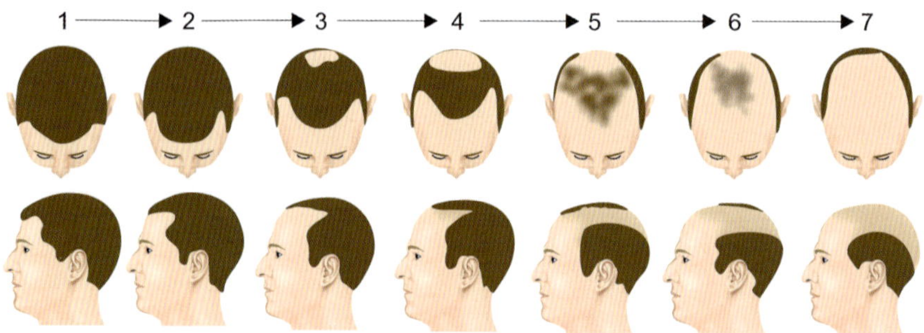

Fig. 112: Men: Alopecia.

- Alopecia areata: Sometimes, the mesotherapy treatment has a benefit effect on the psychosomatic phenomenon which can disappear or be softened.
- Diffuse alopecia: A clear diminution of hair loss can be obtained, with new growth of hair.

Medications used:

- Etamsylate (vasodilator): Stimulation of microcirculation+++
- Vitamin C or polyvitamin solution: Vitamin C Laroscorbine 1G for injection
- Soluvit or Cernevit
- Vitamin H (Biotine), B5 dexpanthenol (Bepanthene)
- Procaine 2%: vector and vasodilatator.

The mixture:

- 10 mL
- Etamsylate: 2 mL = 1 ampule
- Vitamin C or polyvitamined solution: 2 mL
- Vitamin H (Biotin): 1 mL = 1 ampule
- Vitamin B5 dexpanthenol (Bepanthen): 2 mL = 1 ampule
- Procaine 2%: 3 mL.

The material and technique:
- 1 syringe 10 mL
- 1 needle 0.35/4
- I.D.S: Nappage
- Manual or mesogun.

Injection areas:
- Through the hair
- Insist on the most receding areas and on the anterior border of implantation.

Beware the ear pavilions!

Rhythm of the sessions:
- Four sessions to 15 days apart
- Then a maintenance session every 3 months.

Complementary therapies and tips:
- Dietary supplements
- Shampoo treating: Node DS Bioderma
- Do not wash the hair 24 hours following the session
- Do not wash the hair more than twice a week
- Do not cover the hair (hat, turban); hide baldness worsens
- Cut the hair ends; if the hair is very long, it has a stimulating effect on hair growth
- Use a soft brush and detangling.

Results: The hair loss is stopped between the second and the fourth session for more than 90% of patients.

A seborrhea is clearly reduced after three sessions.

Regrowth clearly visible 2 to 3 months after initiation of treatment.

CELLULITE: MESOTHERAPY TREATMENT

The principle of mesotherapy management for cellulite is:

- *Intradermic injections* (very different from subcutaneous or intramuscular injections)
- *A microdosed mixture with*:
  - Vitamin C, thiocolchicoside, and xylocaine
  - Water for injectable preparations (hypotonic, different from physiologic serum or NaCl 9/1,000; the aim—reduce the concentration of the mixture in order to avoid the pain when injecting +++).

We are in the context of lipolysis: stimulating natural elimination by "drainage" of the adipocytes, without destroying them!

(Different from adipocytolysis or adipocyte lysis = destruction of tissues)

Cellulite and Mesotherapy

Mesotherapic drainage with a mixed technique (deep and superficial):

- Deep: 4 mm
- Superficial: 1 or 2 mm
- Antiedematous effect (disinfiltrative) on the derma
- Draining effect (natural stimulation of decreasing number and volume of the adipocytes)
- The effects are *slow and progressive.*

Medications Used

- Water for injectable preparation
- Xylocaine 0.5%: Vasomotor effect and membrane modificator
- Thiocolchicoside:
  - Improves dermal texture and facilitates its restructuration
  - Myorelaxant
  - Defibrosing effect on fibrous cellulite:
    - Activation of TG lipase, lipid oxidation
    - Activation of hormonosensitive lipase
    - Cystein-like oxidating effect.
- Vitamin C injection 1G:
  - Powerful antioxidant
  - Turns pro-collagen into collagen
  - Prevents immunosuppression induced by UVB
  - Prevents excess of melanin formation.

- Trophic effect on collagen, surface smoother
- Lightening effect on pigmented spots
- Stimulating effects on lipolysis
- Etamsylate: Powerful +++
  - Antiedematous
  - Decongestant
  - Vasoactive.

Cellulite (suite)

The mixtures:

- Point by point mesotherapy (IDPC: 4 mm):
  - Xylocaine 0.5%: 1 mL
  - Thiocolchicoside: 1 mL
  - Vitamin C: 2 mL
  - Water for injectable preparation: 6 mL
- Nappage (IED: 1 to 2 mm):
  - Xylocaine 0.5%: 3 mL
  - Thiocolchicoside: 1 mL
  - Vitamin C: 1 mL
  - Etamsylate: 1 mL.

(No water for injectable preparation: the mixture is more hypertonic; Stimulation of the most superficial skin segments, containing the lymphatic system and IED technique, so no pain when injecting)

The material and technique:

- Deep technique (point by point):
  - Needle: 0.35/4 mm
  - IDP (4 mm maximum)
  - Every 0.5 to 1 cm
  - 0.1 cc by punctual injection
  - No more than three 10 mL syringes by session +++.
- Superficial technique (Nappage):
  - Needle: 0.35/4 mm or 0.30/13 mm
  - IDS or epidermic
  - Grid pattern
  - 1 syringe of 6 mL.

Cellulite (suite) (Fig. 113)

The injection areas:

- Deep areas: On fatty deposits
  - Thighs
  - Belly
  - Knees
  - Buttocks
  - Hips.

(Beware: Do not inject on the posterior surface of the arms, even if the patient is asking for—risk of lymphangitis ++++)

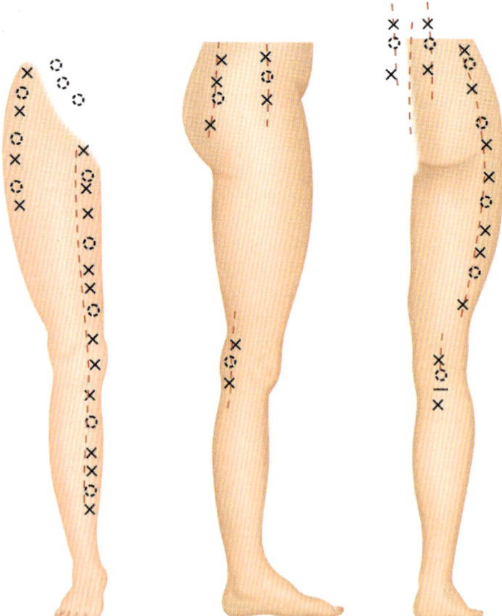

Fig. 113: Cellulitis (Localization of injections).

- Superficial areas: Along the vascular axes of mesodraine, and next to the adipose areas treated.

The rhythm of sessions:

- Four sessions to 8 days apart
- Then four sessions to 15 days apart
- Reminder to 3 months.

Adjuvant treatments:

- Manual lymphatic drainage
- Wearing compression stockings
- Stimulating "sliming" cream
- Nutritional care
- Psychologic support if needed
- Daily physical activity ++++.

14

VASCULAR PATHOLOGY AND MESOTHERAPY

Mesodrain

Physiopathology reminders:

- Venous insufficiency:
- Genetic and hereditary
- Acquired: Post-surgery (stretching, venous slackening, alteration of veno-lymphatic system, lymph node dissection), and pregnancies.
- Risk factors: Tobacco, contraceptive pill, excess weight, sedentarity, sun exposure, and stamping.

Consequences:

- Pain: Heaviness, pain, fatigability, night cramps, tingling, and restless legs.
- Physical consequences:
  - Varicosities, edema, disparition of calf muscle curve, of the ankle's and knee's sculpture ("pole" leg)
  - Obstacle to the venous return, stase, retention
  - Engorgement of the tissues: Risk of an evolution to hydrolipodystrophy (cellulite).

Indications:

- Venous-lymphatic peripheric insufficiency
- Heavy legs, restless legs, and edema of vascular etiology.

[*Important: Eliminate deep venous pathology (Doppler), a cardiac, renal, or neurologic pathology* +++]

Mechanisms:

Stimulation of venous-lymphatic system—from the thoracic canal to the extremities of inferior limbs by:

- Promoting tissues decongestion
- Stimulating drainage
- Fighting against hydrosodic retention.

As usual:

- Clinical record
- Examination
- Eliminate allergy
- General clinic investigation
- Paraclinic research, if necessary.

Medications used:

- Etamsylate: Vasoactive, anti-edema, and decongestant

- Xylocaine 0.5%: Rheologic vector and micro-circulation stimulator
- Calcitonin 100 IU: Analgesic, stimulation, and anti-inflammatory.

The mixture used:
- Calcitonin 100 UI: 1 mL
- Etamsylate: 2 mL
- Xylocaine 0.5%: 2 mL

Injection techniques: Superficial +++
- Intraepidermic (IED), or
- Superficial intradermic: "nappage"

Injection areas: Legs, venous axes: lateral, anterior and posterior, bottom up +++ from the malleolus to the root of the leg.

Rhythm of the injections: D1–D15–D30 in the summer time; on demand

The effects of the treatment: triple effect +++
- Physical effect (cooling effect)
- Mechanic or reflex stimulation (IED or nappage)
- Chemical (drug mixture).

Immediate effect: Cooling effect, pain relief, lightness of the legs, right out the consultation.

Long-term effect: Best comfort during the night sleep, less pains, and less impression of heaviness of the legs during day and night; net decrease of edema, with return to a normal shape of malleolus and carve muscle curve.

So the patients naturally come back every year for a preventive treatment in May and June; there is no more constraint of oral medical treatment.

And, do not forget the associated treatments and prevention:
- Compression stockings
- Avoid stamping
- In the office: Do not cross the legs, footrest
- Avoid wearing high heels
- Avoid: Too hot baths, sun exposure, and ground heating
- Fight against weight excess, risk factors (tobacco, contraceptive pill, sedentarity)
- Regular physic activity: Swimming, walking, bicycle)

(Activate the physiologic pump of the calf muscle)
- Additional treatment with sclerotherapy.

15

DERMATOLOGIC PATHOLOGY AND MESOTHERAPY

Due to the local and locoregional action of mesotherapy, the direct injection of our drugs on the skin area allows us to obtain good results on some dermatologic pathologies.

It can be explained by the extremely stimulating action of our microinjections on the immunocompetent unity, which is very rich and active on the papillary dermis, with optimization of healing processus.

The first consequence is that you have to give priority to superficial injection techniques, particularly the nappage (IDS).

As in all the indications in mesotherapy, the diagnostic step is essential, as the good technique expertise, a rigorous asepsis; we know how the injured skin is susceptible to superinfection.

Treatment of Warts (Fig. 114)

We usually inject thiamine (vitamin B_1) which is efficient on the early stages of lesions:

Mixture: Xylocaine 0.5% 1 mL, vitamin B_1 1 mL

Technique:
- IDP on the plantar warts
- IDS on the other localizations

Rhythm of sessions: J1–J8, every 15 days during the next 2 months.

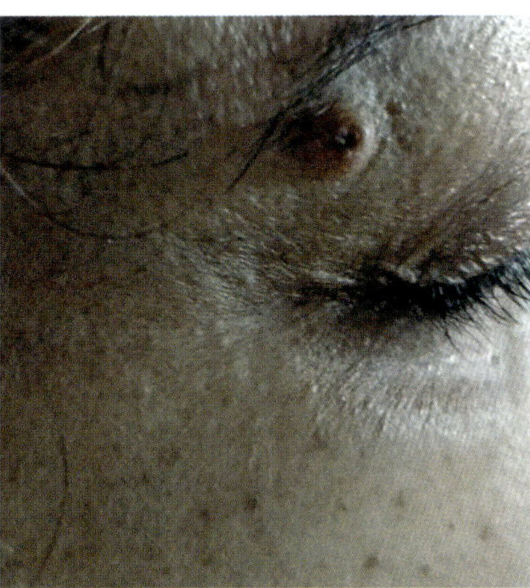

Fig. 114: Warts.

Treatment of Herpes (Fig. 115)

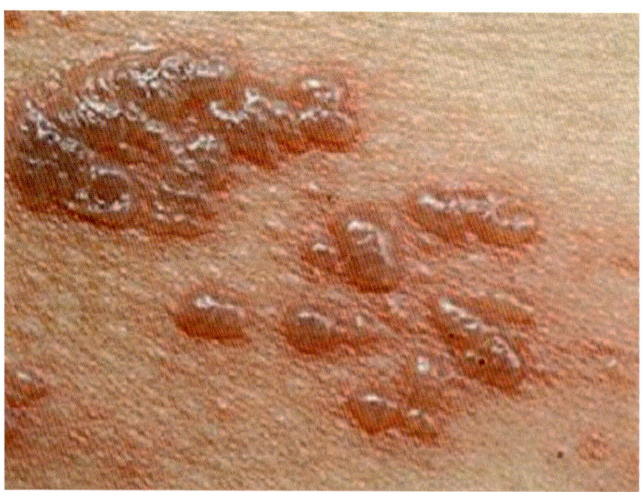

Fig. 115: Herpes.

Treatment of Herpes Thrust

- Mixture 1:
  - Xylocaine 0.5% 1 mL + Acyclovir (200 mg/5 mL) 2 mL
  - Nappage IDS on all vesicles areas.

Associated with:

- Mixture 2:
  - Xylocaine 0.5% 1 mL + Magnesium pidolate 1 mL + Vitamin C 1 mL
  - Nappage IDS or papulas on the ganglionic cervical projections
  - Preauricular and inguinal areas.

Rhythm: J1, J5 to J7

Note: In all the cases, do not carry the virus on a healthy skin; you will have to change the needle before pricking on healthy area.

Prevention of Recurrences

- The mixture: The principle is to maintain a good local, regional, and general immunostimulation; you can use two kinds of mixtures:
  - Xylocaine 0.5% 1 mL, Magnesium pidolate 1 mL, vitamin C 1 mL
  - Physiologic solution (Lavoisier) 9 mL + 0.5 mL influenza vaccine dose.

Use 1 mL of that second mixture.

- The technique: IDS on the recurrences areas; IDS or papulas on the ganglionic cervical projections; always change the needle to prick on healthy skin.
- Rhythm: Every 3 months during 1 to 2 years.

The Treatment of Zona (Fig. 116)

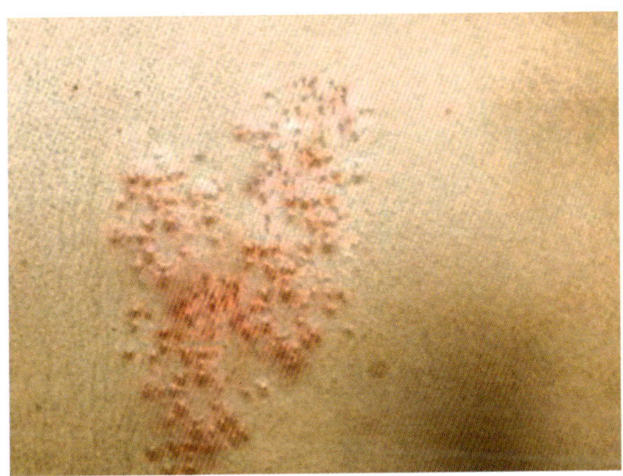

Fig. 116: Zona.

Initial Phase (J1–J3)

- Mixture 1: Xylocaine 0.5% 1 mL + Acyclovir (200 mg/5 mL) 2 mL; IDS nappage on the vesicles areas
- Mixture 2: Xylocaine 0.5% 1 mL + Magnesium pidolate 1 mL, + Vitamin C1 mL; IDS nappage on the whole metamere
- Rhythm J1–J3.

Treatment of Zona between J3 and J7

- Next to the first two sessions or during the first consultation
- The mixture: Analgesic and healing in order to limit the post-herpetic neuralgia; magnesium pidolate 1 mL + vitamin B1 (Bevitine) 1 mL + vitamin B_{12} 1 mL
- Technique: IDS on the whole metamere; always change needle when you treat on healthy skin.
- Rhythm: Two sessions J3–J7.

Treatment of Post-herpetic Neuralgia, Late Phase

- Mixture: Magnesium pidolate 1 mL, Amitriptyline 1 mL or Tiapridal 1 mL and magnesium pidolate 1 mL, vitamin B_1 (Bevitine), vitamin B_{12} 1 mL
- Technique: IDS on the painful metamere
- Rhythm: J1, J8, J15, then J30, J45, and then every 1 or 2 months.

Treatment of Acne

We know now that the formation of retentional lesions, secondary to the proliferation, and the differentiation of keratinocytes is under the influence of the activation of cytokines.

Our mixtures will at aim anti-cytokine.

Moderate Acne

- Mixture 1: Xylocaine 0.5% 1 mL + Magnesium pidolate 1 mL + Vitamin C 1 mL; Nappage IDS on the whole vesicles area associated with:
- Mixture 2: Xylocaine 0.5% 1 mL + Magnesium pidolate 1 mL + Vitamin H 1 mL
- Technique: IDS on acne lesions
- Rhythm: J1, J8, J15, and then every 15 days.

Superinfected Acne

- Mixture: Xylocaine 0.5% 1 mL, magnesium pidolate 1 mL + Cloxacillin (Orbenin)
- Technique: IDS on the acne lesions
- Rhythm: Only one session, then go on with the protocol of moderate acne.

Acne Scars

- Mixture: Silanol salicylate (Conjonctyl) 2 mL + Magnesium pidolate 2 mL
- Technique: Micropapules in the scars
- Rhythm: J1, J8, J15, and then monthly.

Treatment of Eczema (Fig. 117)

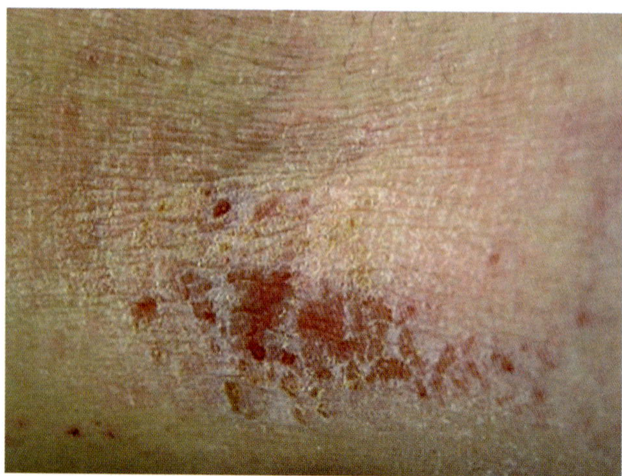

Fig. 117: Eczema.

Treatment of Eczema Thrust

- Mixture: Hydroxyzine (Atarax) or Dexchlorpheniramine (Polaramine) 1 mL + Magnesium pidolate + Vitamin C 1 mL +/- Vitamin A 1 mL if scratching lesions
- Technique: IDS on the lesions of eczema
- Rhythm: J1–J7

Treatment of Chronic Eczema on Dry Skin

- Mixture: Hydroxyzine (Atarax) 1 mL + Magnesium sulfate (Spasmag) 1mL + Vitamin C 1mL

In case of a context of stress, associate the NDV protocol.

- Technique: IDS with large grids on the lesions of eczema
- Rhythm: J1, J7, J21, till disparition of the lesions, and in every recurrence.

Treatment of Psoriasis (Fig. 118)

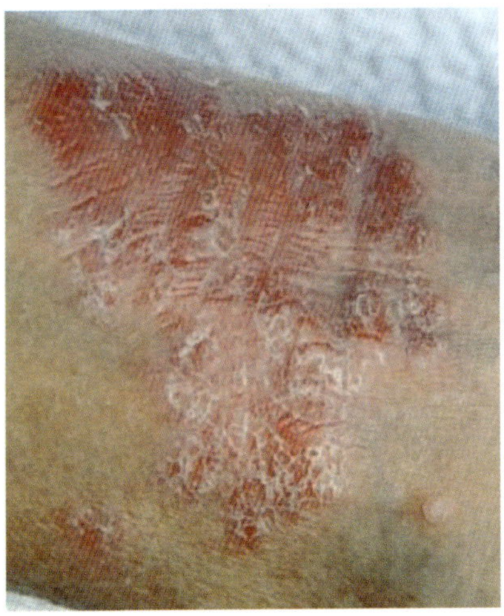

Fig. 118: Psoriasis.

The treatment of psoriasis must be applied only in psoriasis thrusts, respecting Dr Pistor's formula—"few, rarely, on the right place"; if only one session stops the thrust, there is no need for another session.

- Mixture 1—acute phase, first session: Hydroxyzine (Atarax) 1 mL, magnesium pidolate 1 mL, and vitamin C 1 mL
- Mixture 2—chronic phase, second session: Magnesium pidolate 2 mL + Vitamin D 1 mL
- Technique: IDS on the psoriatic lesions
- Rhythm: J1, J8, +/- J14.

In case of a context of stress, associate the NDV protocol.

Treatment of Atopic Dermatitis

Atopic dermatitis is a chronic inflammatory disease of the skin in which formation of free radicals is involved.

Iron has a catalytic role in formation of those activated oxygen forms, and the ascorbic acid allows their elimination.

Lévèque and Al have demonstrated in a study that the derm coming from atopic dermatitis showed higher iron concentrations (44.3 +/– 4.6

mug/L) compared to controls (21.2 +/– 1.8 mug/L), as well significant low concentrations of ascorbic acid (46.7 +/–0.6 versus 176.8 +/– 14.5 mug/L).

Those results suggest that the dermic iron and ascorbic acid levels could be indicators of tissues inflammation, and could be involved in dermatologic diseases like atopic dermatitis.

- Mixture: Magnesium pidolate 1 mL + Vitamin C 1 mL
- Technique: IDS with large grids on the lesions
- Rhythm: J1, J8, J15, J21.

16

MESOLIFT

History

Mesotherapy was invented by Dr Michel Pistor (1952). The anti-radical mesotherapy has been developed later by Dr André Dalloz Bourguignon in the eighties.

Mesolift appeared in the end of the nineties with the arrival of the nonreticulated hyaluronic acids.

Nowadays, there exists a plethoric offer of products, protocols, and techniques.

Mesolift Definition

This is a technique of facial rejuvenation, used in prevention of skin aging and even its repair. The product or the mixture is homogeny, logical, efficient, and can be applied in mesotherapy, that is to say epidermic and intradermic.

We use product which have a legal authorization of marketing or a CE Label!
The aim is to provoke an *intense stimulation of the skin, its regeneration, even its protection.*

The mesolift indication is the correction of skin extrinsic aging. It also allows to treat some superficial wrinkles—"wrinkles of the pillow", malar and infraorbital, jugal wrinkles (accordion folds), and wrinkles of the crow's foot.

Mesolift also improves dull skins, hypotonic, sagged, and dehydrated skins.

Nonindications of Mesolift

Mesolift has no effect on deep wrinkles or skin folds—nasolabial folds, commissural folds, and horizontal folds of the nose's root.
No effect on the spots or acne.

Contraindications of Mesolift

Pregnancy, breast feeding, inflammatory skin areas, and/or infectious (acne, herpes), hypertrophic scars, autoimmune diseases, immunosuppressant treatments, and known sensitivity to hyaluronic acid.

Precautions

- *Patients must not take aspirin, anti-inflammatory treatments, anti-vitamin K, and anticoagulation treatments.*

- *Do not associate with immediate laser treatment, chemical peeling or dermabrasion.*
- *No make up while the 12 hours following the injection.*
- *No solar exposure or UV while the 2 days following the injection.*
- *Good cleansing and skin cleansing.*
- *Disinfection of the skin with a compatible antiseptic.*
- *Preventive treatment of herpes 8 days before and 8 days after the session for risky patients. Double test on risky patients.*

Side Effects of Mesolift

Some effects like bruises or scratches are possible, even if they are rare; sometimes allergic reactions to the injected products can happen.

The Products We Use

- Vasoactive: Magnesium
- Polyvitamins, vitamin C
- Conjonctyl or organic silicium
- Viscoelastic gels.

The Properties of Polyvitamins

- Composition: Vitamins A-D3-E-B_1-B_2-B_5-B_6-B_{12}-PP-C-folic acid-vitamin H
- Antiradical vitaminic action
- Factor of tissue growth: Vitamin A, D3—degenerative and trophic troubles
- Contraindication: Known allergy to vitamin B_1.

The Vitamin

Powerful antiradical effect, associated with organic silicium (healing), and regulation of complexion.

Properties of Silicium (Monoethyl trisilanol orthohydroxybenzoate of sodium)

- Indication: Filling of skin depressions (wrinkles and scars) by intradermic injections.
- Strong healing effect on the conjunctive tissue
- To associate with antiradical products
- Contraindication of salicylate derivatives: Known allergy to aspirin.

Properties of Magnesium

- Fights against oxidative stress
- Fights against fibrosis formation
- Anti-cytokine action and microcirculation stimulation by vasomotor action
- Promotes angiogenesis.

The Hyaluronic Acid: Has properties of viscoelasticity and hydration.

There are three "kinds" of Mesolift:

- Mesolift with pure hyaluronic acid
- Mesolift with hyaluronic acid diluted with vitamins
- Mesolift with pure vitamins.

Mesolift with Pure Hyaluronic Acid (Nonreticulated)

Advantages

- The use of hyaluronic acid in Mesolift allows to compensate the loss of endogen hyaluronic acid.
- The hyaluronic acid injected reaches quickly the derm; it occurs a recolonization of the extracellular matrix (fibroblasts).
- The product is preconditioned for the realization of the injection, avoiding extemporaneous mixture.

Disadvantage

- The cost is higher.

Clinical Results

- Clear improvement of skin elasticity and hydration; improvement of fine lines; best firmness and homogeneous skin.
- More fair and shiny complexion.
- Formation of a protecting shield against free radicals.

Technique

The hyaluronic acid is injected in the superficial area of the derm; microinjections will be done, 2 mm papules with parallel lines with spots distant from few mm to 1 cm.

According to the type of skin, some papules can still be apparent 2 or 3 days after a session.

After the treatment, the skin should be massed in order to spread the product and "smash" the papules.

The treatment protocol and the rhythm of the sessions depend on the aging stage:

Many sessions can be necessary till the desired effect is obtained, 2 to 3 sessions with 1 month interval, then a session every 6 months. Keeping this effect will be guaranteed by a regular maintenance. If needed, this treatment can be completed by injections for filling wrinkles.

Pre-injection advice: If the pores are dilated, it is advised to make a preparation with alpha-hydroxy acids (AHAs) or acid vitamin A, 2 or 3 days before.

Mesolift with Hyaluronic Acid and Vitamins

Advantages

Double action: Rehydration and protection against aging of the skin (anti-radical, growth factors). The mixture is easier to inject (more fluid) if a good technique is applied.

Disadvantage

Needs more initial sessions for a good result.

The treatment protocol and the rhythm of the sessions depend on the aging stage:

- Many sessions can be necessary till you can get the effect you wish.
- One session every 15 days during 2 months, then a session every 2 to 4 months.
- A minimum time limit of 15 days should be applied between two sessions.
- Keeping this result will be guaranteed by a regular maintenance.

Mesolift with Vitamins

Advantages: Has a good effect on the skin complexion (shining effect); it has an antiradical effect, stimulates the growth factors (vitamins A and D, and silicium) and the puncture.

It is easy to do, and low-cost.

Disadvantages: Less rehydrating; the sessions must be at close intervals to obtain a good result; obligation to use preconditioned mixtures.

Magnesium: 2 cc
Organic silicium: 2 cc
Vitamin C 1G: 2 cc

Technique

IDS (nappage) or IED on the whole face, including the buccal contour, the crow's feet, the cleavage, and the hands. Make more or less tight lines, depending on the area we have to treat. The frequency of sessions: every 15 days in the first 2 months, then once a month the next 3 months, and then every 2 months for maintenance.

The results can be improved by application of vitamin C in topical application.

Important skin stimulation; the procedure is painless. There is rapid action. The treated areas are wider.

Conclusion

Mesolift is a basic care in the therapeutic arsenal of aesthetic medicine. It is the intermediary between cosmetic cares and heavier healing techniques. The diversity of products allows it to fit to the skin degree of degradation, to the care program proposed.

17

SCARS

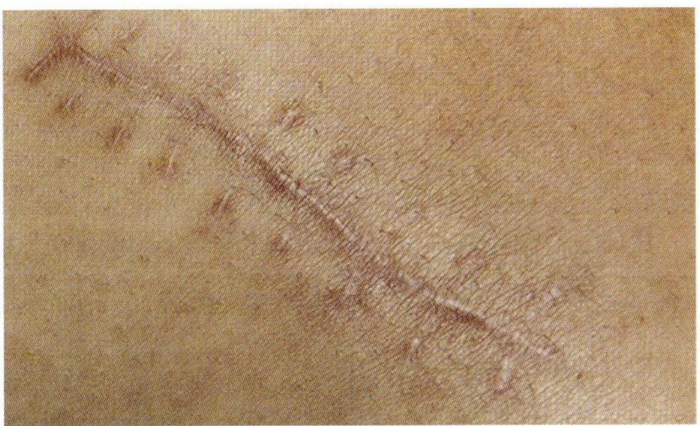

Fig. 119: Scars.

Definition

Traumatic or surgical, stitched wound either not, dating from 4 days to several years, in evolutionary phase of healing, or in phase of ending scar, with esthetic or functional after-effects (Fig. 119).

Physiopathology

There are four phases:
Phase 1: Hemostasis (Day 1)
Phase 2: Inflammation (Day 1 to 4)
Phase 3: Proliferation-granulation-contraction (Day 4 to 21)
Phase 4: Remodeling-maturation (Day 21 to 2 years)

The mesotherapic treatment is applied from the third phase, scrupulously respecting the rules of disinfection of the skin in the post-surgery period.

Clinical Examination

- *Aesthetic disorders:* Recessed tissues, embossed tissues, atonic, thin, thick, hyperkeratotic, pigmented, unpigmented, white, blue, purple, red, hot, cold, hypervascularized, and hypovascularized.
- *Functional disorders:* Adherence to deep planes, retraction, lack of suppleness while moving, hypoesthesia, hyperesthesia, and dysesthesia.
- Finesse touch, with the fingertips, by stretching or pushing, and by pinching skin softly.
- Exploration of the adjacent areas and of underlying organs.
- Look for a locoregional disorder.

Additional tests are often useless.

The Mesotherapic Treatment

Techniques

- IED epidermal, IDS Nappage, with lines spaced to 2–3 millimeters.
- Papules: IDP point by point.

Main Mixtures

J4—post-surgery scar:
- Lidocaine 1%: 2 cc
- Etamsylate: 2 cc
- Vitamin C: 2 cc.

J4 to 2 years scar:
- Lidocaine 1%: 2 cc
- Etamsylate: 2 cc
- • Vitamin C: 2 cc.

Ancient scar with burning sensation:
- Lidocaine 1%: 2 cc
- Magnesium pidolate: 2 cc
- Vitamin C: 2 cc.

Ancient and painful scar:
- Lidocaine 1%: 2 cc
- Magnesium pidolate: 2 cc
- Vitamin C: 2 cc
- Salmon calcitonin 100 IU: 1 cc.

Application areas: On the scar, far beyond the area.

Rhythm: D1-D7-D14-D30

Associations:
- Laser: Mainly the ablative lasers, dermabrasion by CO Laser, or Erbium-Yag, in order to smooth the ancient and thick scars.
- Carboxytherapy: CO_2 epidermal injections in order to decrease the inflammation look of the scar.

Note: It is possible to apply a mesotherapic treatment from the 4th post-surgery day, scrupulously respecting the rules of disinfection of the skin, and using exclusively the epidermal IED technique which does not cross the basal layer.

With the same precautions, it is possible to treat a scar next to a prosthesis area (e.g. a knee prosthesis).

The mixture of the drugs used depends of the clinical examination findings, without forgetting the general state of the patient, and is adapted to every scar.

The scars, even very ancient, often keep a strong reactive potential.

Mesotherapy is a technique of choice for restoring good local conditions of growth tissue.

Only the recent keloid scars are moderately receptive to mesotherapy.

18

KELOID

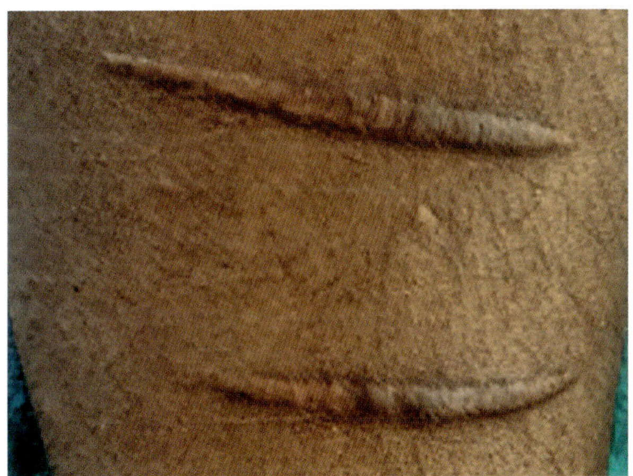

Fig. 120: Keloid.

Definition

Fibrous scar formation, making an inesthetic, more or less voluminous roll, more often after a surgical wound (or any other wound) (Fig. 120).

Physiopathology

Dysregulation of the healing—fibrosis process.

Mesotherapic Treatment

- Bleomycin (1 fl)
- Procaine: 2 cc
- Pentoxifylline: 2 cc
- Salmon Calcitonin 100 IU: 1 cc

Technique

Epidermal (IDS).

STRETCH MARKS

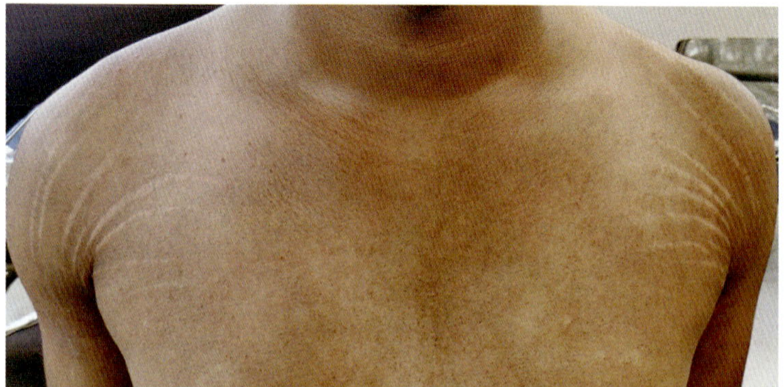

Fig. 121: Stretch marks.

Definition

Linear dermis atrophy, well-delimitated, and covered with wrinkled epidermis; they are in preference located on the abdomen (periumbilical area), breasts, buttocks, condylar areas of the thighs, and lumbosacral area (Fig. 121).

Stretch marks appear on the place where the skin is subject to excessive strains (breast, abdomen, thighs, hips, lower back, shoulders, and arms). Their colors may vary from red for the most recent stretch marks, to white for the oldest.

Other causal factors in the formation of stretch marks are identified: hereditary anomalies of the conjunctive tissues, excessive adrenocortical activity, and intense sportive practice, especially among the culturists.
Another factor: The cream with anti-depigmenting action.

Predisposing Factors

- Pregnancy
- Obesity
- Horizontal growth of dorsolumbar, hips, and thigh areas
- Sport activity
- Medical treatments (local and general corticotherapy).

Mesotherapic Treatment

Indications

- The recent stretch marks are always a good indication.
- All the localizations, except abdomen can be treated during pregnancy.
- Abdominal stretch marks will be treated exclusively in postpartum.

Modalities

- First mixture
  - Lidocaine 1%: 1 mL
  - Magnesium pidolate: 2 mL
  - Cernevit (Polyvitamin mixture): 2 mL
  - Technique: IDS + IDP on stretch mark, and around I healthy skin.
- Second mixture:
  - Lidocaine 1% : 1 mL
  - Conjonctyl: 3 mL (or NTCF 135 2 mL).

Technique

Retrograde injection under the stretchmark, with a needle 0.29 × 13 mm, under the colored area.

Area

Prick on the stretchmark, overflowing widely on healthy skin, and with the second mixture.

Rhythm of the sessions: J0, J15, J30, J45, J60, and J90.

Complementary Treatment

- On recent stretch marks: Vitamin A acid 0.005 cream, vascular laser Nd: YAG 1064 nm, which stimulates the formation of collagen fibers. Carboxytherapy: vasodilatation and stimulation of collagen production.
- On ancient stretch marks:
  - Fractioned ablative laser on clear skins
  - 2 to 4 sessions
  - Fractioned non-ablative laser
  - LED + Radiofrequency.

There is a real benefit of mesotherapy sessions on the recent stretch marks; we have to admit the limits of our treatment on ancient stretch marks, knowing they are a healing modality.

CONCLUSION

To conclude this book, let me hope that it will bring to our young students and colleagues a useful and practical tool in their daily practice.

To me, mesotherapy gave me many satisfactions, as well to my patients, thanks to the main qualities of this method:

- Safe, with rare side effects
- Economic
- Easy to practice
- Efficient

The development of teaching of mesotherapy in many countries, with the natural requirement and seriousness of this discipline, is a guarantee for the practitioners who could be interested to add this technique to their practice.

BIBLIOGRAPHY

1. Bourguignon D. La Mésothérapie. Paris: Maloine Editeur; 1983.
2. Coulon JH. Stimulothérapies Comparées en pratique médicale. Paris: Maloine Editeur; 1987.
3. Coulon JH. Approche mésothérapique dans le traitement de la Dystonie Neuro-Végétative, à propos de 100 cas; 1985.
4. Inter-University Diploma of Aesthetic Mesotherapy (French Diploma of Mesotherapy), Paris, 2015. Dr Labenne, Dr Salato, Dr Taffin
5. Jean-Claude P. Congrès de Rome 1982 : Les Dystonies neuro-végétatives en mésothérapie-Le traitement des dystonies neuro-végétatives en mésothérapie.
6. Laurens D, Bonnet C, Perrin JJ. Guide pratique de Mésothérapie, 2nd edition. Paris: Elsevier-Masson Editeur; 2012.
7. Le Coz J. Traité de Mésothérapie, 2nd édition. Paris: Masson Editeur; 2009.
8. Malige Y, Saint-Hillier S. Enseignements du CERM de Franche-Comté.
9. Perrin JJ. Les différentes techniques d'injection en mésothérapie ; enseignement du 24 Septembre 2008, Faculté de Médecine de la Pitié Salpêtrière.
10. Pistor M. Mésothérapie, un défi thérapeutique. Paris: Maloine Editeur; 1982.

INDEX

Page numbers followed by *f* refer to figure

A

Acetic salicylic acid 72
Achilles
  tendinitis 67
  tendon rupture 67
Acid 81
Acne
  moderate 92
  scars 92
  superinfected 92
  treatment of 91
Acouphenes 37, 37*f*
Acrocyanosis 29
Acroparesthesia 29
Acrosyndromes 29, 30*f*
Acupan 73
Acupuncture 35, 73
Adrenalin 14
Aerogastria 30, 31*f*
Aerophagy 30
Algodystrophy 14, 31, 31*f*
Alkaline 81
Allergy 14, 28, 32, 77
Allopathic drugs 13
Alopecia 32, 33, 79, 82*f*
  areata 79, 81, 82
  classification of 79
  diffuse 79, 80
  mesotherapic management of 81
  various stages of 80*f*
Alpha-hydroxy acids 97
Anafranil 13, 41
Androgenic alopecia 79, 82
Ankle, sprain of 65, 65*f*
Antalgic drugs 72
Anthralin 81
Antiallergic medications 37
Anti-arthrosis medications 35, 73
Antibiotics 14
Anticoagulants 81
Antidepressants 81
Anti-inflammation drugs 74
Anxiety 14, 33
Arnica 14, 65, 72
Arnold's nerve 54*f*
Arnold's neuralgia 54, 55*f*
Arteriovenous system 5
Arteritis 14, 33, 34*f*, 72
Arthrosis 14, 34, 39
Aspirin 72
Asthenia 35
Asthma 32, 36
Atarax 13
Atopic dermatitis, treatment of 93
Avlocardyl 53

B

Back pain 14, 59
Bacterial infection, acute 77
Bepanthene 32, 82
Biotin 13, 32, 82
Bleomycin 101
Blood pressure, treatments 81
Bone
  fracture 59
  metastases 72*f*
Brain pain management system 71*f*
Bronchodilators 37
Bruises 28
Burn 81

C

Calcaneal spur 66
Calcitonin 13, 29, 32, 33, 35, 37, 43, 45, 49-51, 59, 61, 62, 64, 68, 73, 74, 88
Calcium 44
Cancerology 72
Carcinoma, basocellular 81
Cardiovascular disorder, severe 77
Carotids 37
Cataract 37, 38*f*
Cellular structure 5
Cellulite 75, 84, 85
  treatment 22
Cellulitis 86*f*
Cephalalgia 38, 52
Cerebral circulation, insufficiency of 48, 48*f*
Cernevit 82
Cervical
  arthrosis 38, 39
  origin, headache of 38
  rachis, arthrosis of 34
  spine 39
Cervicodynia 38, 38*f*
Christmas tree 30
Chronology 1
Cicatricial
  alopecia 81
  pemphigoid 81

Coccydynia 39, 39*f*
Colic 40*f*
  hepatic 40, 40*f*
  nephric 40, 40*f*
Colopathy 40, 40*f*
Complex regional pain syndrome 14
Constipation 40
Contact sensibilization, induction of 81
Corticoids 14, 81
  inhaled 37
Corticotherapy 102
Coxarthrosis 34, 41*f*
Cramp 41, 41*f*
Cruralgia 51
Cryotherapy, sequela of 81
Cyclosporine A 81
Cyst, synovial 65, 65*f*, 66, 66*f*
Cytostatics 81

D

Danazol 80
Depression 41
Dexpanthenol 82
Diabetes 27, 81
Dibutyl squaric acid 81
Diclofenac 39, 43, 45, 60
Diphencyprone 81
Diphenylcyclopropenone 81
Disinfection, products for 12, 13
Dorsal rachis, arthrosis of 34
Dry mesotherapy 23, 23*f*, 25, 47, 47*f*
Dry puncture 46
Dry skin 93
Dysmenorrhea 42, 42*f*
Dyspepsia 42, 43
Dysplasia, ectodermic 81
Dystonia, neurovegetative 33, 53, 53*f*

E

Ears, humming of 37
Eczema 92*f*, 93
  treatment of 92
Elbow 45, 45*f*
  hygroma of 46*f*
Endorphins 4
Enzyme 5
Epicondylitis 14, 43, 43*f*
Epidermic nevus 81
Epidermis 75
  lifting of 76
Epidermodermal junction 76
Epigastralgia 28
Epilepsy 77
Epiphysitis 44, 44*f*
Esberiven 49, 52, 61
Etamsylate 13, 29, 33, 35, 37, 43, 45, 49-53, 55, 57, 61, 62, 64, 65, 67, 68, 72-74, 82, 85, 88
Extracellular matrix 4

F

Facial
  and trigeminal nerve neuralgia 54, 55, 57
  rejuvenation 21
Farsightedness 61
Fibrosis 101
Fibrous cellulite 84
Fibrous scar formation 101
Flexor tendon sheath 65

G

Gastralgia 44, 44*f*
Gate control system 71*f*
Gauze-cotton wool 77
Genetic disease 81
Golden salts 14
Gonarthrosis 34

H

Hair loss 79
  management 75
Hallux valgus 44, 44*f*
Headache 38, 72
Healing, dysregulation of 101
Height over time, loss of 59
Hemicrania 72
Hepatitis 81
Herpes 90*f*
  simplex virus 77
  treatment of 90
  zoster 68
Hips
  arthrosis of 34
  osteoarthritis of 41
Homeopathy 35, 73
  drugs 14
Hormone, adrenocorticotropic 80
Hyaluronic acid 97, 98
Hydrosodic retention, fighting against 87
Hydrosol polyvit 35
Hygroma 45, 45*f*
Hyperplasia, adrenal 80
Hyperthyroidism 81
Hypophyseal dysfunction 80
Hypothyroidism 81

I

Immunostimulation 7*f*, 46, 46*f*, 47*f*
Impingement syndrome 59
Inflammation, acute period of 43, 45
Inflammatory skin condition, acute 77
Influenza 81

Injections
    localization of 30*f*, 31*f*, 33*f*, 34, 36*f*-44*f*, 46*f*, 48*f*-53*f*, 55*f*, 57*f*, 60*f*-66*f*, 68*f*, 69*f*, 72*f*, 86*f*
    techniques of 19, 25*f*
Insomnia 47, 48*f*
Intraepidermal injection 21*f*
Intraepidermic technique 26*f*

K

Keloid 101, 101*f*
Ketoprofen 74
Knee 45, 45*f*
    arthrosis 34, 50, 50*f*
        radiography 50*f*
    synovial cyst of 66*f*

L

Laroxyl 13
Leishmaniasis 81
Leprosy 81
Lichen planus 81
Linear dermis atrophy 102
Lipothymic reaction 28
Little pain 22
Loco dolente 27
Low molecular weight heparin 14
Lower limbs
    arteriopathy 33
    insufficiency of venous circulation of 49, 49*f*
Lumbago 51, 74
Lumbar and sacrum, arthrosis of 34
Lymph node dissection 87
Lymphatic drainage, manual 86

M

Magnesium 30, 32, 34-36, 38-41, 50, 51, 53, 63-65, 67, 68, 72-74, 96
    pidolate 13
    properties of 96
Mastodynia 52, 52*f*
Melanin formation, prevents excess of 84
Mesalyse 11, 11*f*
Mesodrain 87
Mesoflash 10, 10*f*
Mesogun 2*f*, 10, 10*f*, 77
    disinfection of 12*f*
Mesolift 75, 95, 97, 98
    contraindications of 95
    nonindications of 95
    side effects of 96
Mesoperfusion 25
Mesotherapic treatment 100, 101, 103
Mesotherapy 1, 14, 19, 70, 72, 75, 79, 84, 87
    aesthetic 77
    basic kit for 8*f*
    consultation 27
    epidermic 20, 20*f*, 25
    equipment 8
    etymology of 1
    fundamental studies in 2
    history of 1
    kits 9
    medicines used in 13
    punctual systematized 24
    rules of pharmacology in 6
    side effects of 28
    studies in 2
    techniques 20
    treatment 84
    vascular action of 6
Metabolic disorder, severe 77
Meteorism 30
Microcirculation 67
Migraine 13, 14, 38, 52, 52*f*
Monoethyl trisilanol orthohydroxybenzoate 96
Muscle contraction 74
Muscular cramps 41
Mycobacteria infection 28, 28*f*
Myorelaxant 13, 72, 84

N

Nappage 76, 76*f*, 85
Nausea 42
Necrosis, cutaneous 28
Needle
    destruction 11*f*
    fear of 27
    inclination of 21*f*
    proper action of 4
    syringe 8
    types of 8, 8*f*
Nefopam chlorhydrate 73
Nepanthen 13
Nerves
    greater occipital 55
    lesser occipital 55
    trigeminal 55*f*, 56*f*
Neuralgia 54
    intercostal 54, 57, 57*f*
    occipital 55
    trigeminal 56, 57*f*
    types of 55
Neuralgic system 54*f*
Nutritional care 86
Nutritional deficiency 81

O

Obesity 102
Oligotherapy 35, 73
Organic silicium 14, 96
Osteoporosis 14, 58, 58*f*
Ovarian hyperplasia 80

P

Pain 14, 28, 70
- acute 72
- chronic 55, 72
- dermatologic 72
- management 54, 70
- metastatic 72
- neurologic 72, 73
- neuropathic 72, 73
- rheumatologic 72, 73
- tracks 70
- treatments 72
- vascular 72
- visceral 72

Papular depth 22*f*
Papular technique 22, 22*f*
Papule 25
Pentoxifylline 101
Peptic ulcer disease 17*f*
Periarthritis 59
- scapulohumeral 59

Pharmacokinetics 6*f*
Phloroglucinol 13, 30, 40, 42, 72
Physiotherapy 35, 73
Pigmentation disorders 77
Piroxicam 13
Polaramine 32, 36, 63
- antiallergic 13

Polycystic ovaries syndrome 80
Polyvitamin 96
- properties of 96
- solution 82

Post-herpetic neuralgia, treatment of 91
Powerful antioxidant 84
Pregnancy 27, 77, 102
Presbycusis 60, 60*f*
Presbyopia 61, 61*f*
Procaine 82, 101
Profenid 34, 50, 51, 64, 68, 73
Progesterone 80
Propranolol 13
Psoralen and ultraviolet A therapy 81
Psoriasis 93*f*
- treatment of 93

Pure hyaluronic acid 97

R

Radiodermitis 81
Raynaud's disease 29, 62, 62*f*
Raynaud's phenomenon 62
Raynaud's syndrome 62
Rheumatology 14
Rhinitis 32, 63, 63*f*
- allergic 63

Rhizarthrosis 63, 64, 64*f*
- radiography 63*f*

Rivotril 13

S

Salmon calcitonin 101
Salmon origin 13
Sarcoidosis 81
Scalp mesotherapy 79*f*
Scapula
- periarthritis of 59*f*, 60*f*
- presbyopia of 61*f*

Scarring alopecia 79, 81
Scars 75, 99, 99*f*
- hypertrophic 77

Scheuermann disease 44
Sciatica 51
Silicium, properties of 96
Sinusitis 64, 64*f*
Skin
- different depths of 26*f*
- major stimulation of 22
- stimulation of 75
- structure 4, 4*f*, 19*f*

Slow mesoperfusion 24, 24*f*
Sodium, monoethyl trisilanol orthohydroxybenzoate of 96
Soluvit 44, 82
Spasfon 13, 72
Spinal cord 42
Sports
- activity 102
- injuries 14, 72, 74, 74*f*
- traumatology 74

Sprain 14, 65*f*
Steroids, anabolic 80
Stratum corneum 7*f*
Stretch marks 75, 102, 102*f*
Superficial technique 85
Syphilis 81

T

Talalgia 66, 66*f*
Tendinitis 14, 67, 67*f*, 68*f*, 74
Tendon, healing of 67
Tennis elbow 43
Terbutaline 13, 32
Testosterone 80
Tetracemate, injection of 60
Thiamine 13
Thiocolchicoside 13, 32, 34, 35, 38, 41, 42, 47, 50, 51, 54, 55, 59, 68, 69, 73, 74, 84, 85
Thompson test 67, 67*f*
Thrombophlebitis 16*f*
Thumb, Z-shaped deformation of 64
Tic douloureux 56
Tofranil 41
Trimebutine 42, 44
Tuberculosis 81
Tumors, carcinoid 80
Typhus 81

V

Vascular pathology 75, 87
Venolymphatic system, alteration of 87
Venous insufficiency 14, 72, 87
Venous lymphatic peripheric insufficiency 87
Viral infection 77
Viscoelastic gels 96
Vitamin 35, 73, 96, 98
  A 92
  B_1 13
  B_{12} 14, 55, 57, 69, 73
  B_5 dexpanthenol 82
  B_6 13
  C 13, 82, 84, 85, 96
    injection 84
    laroscorbine 82
  D 93
  E 14
  H 82

W

Waldeyer area 36*f*, 47
Warts 89*f*
  treatment of 89

X

Xylocaine 29, 30, 32-47, 49-55, 57, 59-65, 67-69, 73, 84, 85, 88

Z

Zona 68, 68*f*, 69*f*, 72, 72*f*, 81, 91*f*
  treatment of 91